...mapped Mind

Christian Donlan is an award-winning journalist whose work has appeared in the *New Statesman*, *Edge* magazine and *Vice*, among other publications. He is a features editor at Eurogamer.net. He lives in Brighton with his family.

The Unmapped Mind

A Memoir of Neurology, Multiple
Sclerosis and Learning How to Live

CHRISTIAN DONLAN

PENGUIN BOOKS

PENGUIN BOOKS

UK | USA | Canada | Ireland | Australia
India | New Zealand | South Africa

Penguin Books is part of the Penguin Random House group of companies
whose addresses can be found at global.penguinrandomhouse.com.

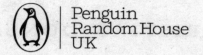

First published by Viking 2018
Published in Penguin Books 2019
001

The publisher is grateful for permission to reprint the following:
extract from *Carter Beats the Devil* by Glen David Gold on page vii,
copyright © Glen David Gold, 2001. Reproduced by permission
of Hodder and Stoughton Limited; and lines from *The Waste Land*
on page 239, copyright © *The Waste Land* by T. S. Eliot, Faber and Faber Ltd

Printed and bound in Great Britain by Clays Ltd, Elcograf S.p.A.

A CIP catalogue record for this book is available from the British Library

ISBN: 978-0-241-98093-4

www.greenpenguin.co.uk

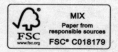

Penguin Random House is committed to a
sustainable future for our business, our readers
and our planet. This book is made from Forest
Stewardship Council® certified paper.

To Sarah, Leon, Jonathan and Leonora,
with love and boundless gratitude.

'There were never moments in your life when you actually saw something end, for whether you knew it or not something else was always flowering. Never a disappearance, always a transformation.'

Glen David Gold, *Carter Beats the Devil* (2001)

'When a patient calls on you, he is under no obligation to have a simple disease just to please you.'

Jean-Martin Charcot (15 November 1887)

Contents

1. The Inland Empire

I have never really liked the fact that I have a brain. The thought of it has always made me feel vulnerable and compromised and delicate, as if I were walking around with a glass of water balanced on my head, waiting for it to spill. And I now suspect that I am not entirely alone in this. When, recently, my daughter, Leon, first became aware of her own brain – when she first noticed the presence of her thoughts sounding inside her head – she assumed she was unwell.

One evening a few weeks back, I was drawn through the house by sudden sobbing. After I'd found Leon crying in the living room, and after I'd wiped her nose and pinned back her hair, she told me, with much floundering and fumbling to get the meaning out, that she had pictures stuck in her head and she didn't know why.

The pictures made her happy, she said. They were mainly pictures of Lego bricks, cluttered and colourful, spread across the floor of the living room. But she didn't understand where these pictures had come from, and they didn't seem to be going anywhere in a hurry. Now she was scared that she would always have pictures of Lego bricks stuck in her head. I think she even worried there might be a real brick or two lodged in there.

Leon was nearly four by the time of this revelation, and as soon as she understood that the pictures were called thoughts, and that thoughts are a very normal kind of magic, we decided to conquer this new information in the most direct manner we could both imagine. I sketched the basic perimeter on a piece of paper, and then my daughter took twenty minutes to draw a map of the kind of landscape that this book explores. It's a map of the interior of the skull, a map of the beautiful, maddening, difficult place that thoughts come from. Except, because she was nearly four, the picture Leon drew is filled with features that do not appear in most neurological textbooks. There is a lot of lava inside her skull, apparently, and at least one waterfall. There are a surprising number of ponies knocking about too.

I was not surprised that this map helped to calm her down. When I was young, maps and stories were inseparable. Every book I read seemed to come with an outline of the territory that it covered laid out across the endpapers, and every atlas I owned was dense with little figures and scenes waiting to explain the history of an island or to give shape and weight to the science throbbing away beneath the pale surface of an ocean. The adventures I liked did not always require opposition – I was a nervous child and easily frightened – but they did require a journey, a sense of movement through a landscape cluttered with strange, promising names and the suggestion of sights that might be worth a visit.

A map is an adventure, but if you are nervous and easily frightened it is also a comfort. I could look at the map before reading a book and get a sense of the kinds of elements it would contain – the rough shape of the story, and perhaps a limit to its potential to scare me. Maps were a means of fixing things in place and making them safe.

An obvious question emerges from this, and I have been turning it over for the last few years. What does it mean to explore a terrain that resists most attempts to document it? What does it mean to find yourself without a map?

I know a few places like this, I think, and one of them is intimately bound up with Leon and those Lego bricks. Since the early days of our relationship, whenever the weekend came around, with Sarah still sleeping, Leon and I would get up together and head to the living room, where we would upend the Lego box. We would listen to that great collapsing splash that Lego creates when it moves en masse and then, Leon balanced in my lap, I would build. We would build. One piece connecting to another. Toys she was far too young for and I was far too old for. Toys that were suddenly perfect for both of us.

In my memory, this ritual started just months after Leon was born, as soon as she entered that glorious age when every experience is worth having. Your job, as a child, is to have no job. Your job as a child is to be roving eyes and roving hands. The world is a thing to be examined closely, and then it is a thing to be grasped. Our time with the living-room Lego feels idyllic when I look back on it now. Maybe it is suspiciously idyllic. Sometimes I will tell this story to someone else and they will raise an eyebrow, unconvinced, and it will dawn on me that what I am telling them is not quite the whole story – that there is a more interesting aspect to our Lego mornings, and I have slowly, steadily, forgotten it.

I have forgotten that, for many months, it was me doing all the building. I think Leon just snoozed at first, strapped into a bouncy chair. As time passed, she would be a warm weight in my lap while my arms reached around her for bricks, her fragile head resting under my chin. Sometimes, she would tap her fingers on her palms with that look of amused indulgence that children often adopt when confronted with the behaviour of adults. And the behaviour she was witnessing is pretty simple for me to decode, frankly. I was Leon's father, but I did not know how to be myself around her. I did not know how to play with her yet, or even if she *could* play at this age. Things did not always come naturally to Leon and me in the early months. The Lego became a thing to do that allowed us to spend time together so we could start to understand each other better.

To put it another way, I met my daughter in a delivery suite at Sussex County Hospital in Brighton, but I got to know her on the floor of the living room in our house, bricks scattered about and a strange landscape shifting around us.

Over the next few years Leon steadily became more involved. She slowly moved from watching to wanting to take part – and finally to leading.

And I started to notice things too. I noticed the flickerings of her tentative nature as she reached for her first bricks and then tried to eat them. I noticed her easy smile and also her unpredictability, discovering that something that would make her laugh one day – clipping bricks around the ribbon of a helium balloon, say, to stop it from floating to the ceiling – would make her sob with fury the next.

Destruction was an early fascination. I would start constructing a building and she would take it to pieces, punching and giggling. It was a race to see who could work more quickly. Eventually, she wanted to put one brick on another herself. Gaining control of her hands and fingers eventually allowed her to twist one piece into the correct position and snap it cleanly into place.

The first time she put two bricks together like this she laughed for a full minute at what she had done. And then she gave herself a week off. The Lego has been like that throughout: a series of revelations for both of us. Simple blocks, and yet we use them to make endless tumbledown cities and bizarre, craggy mountain ranges that fragment into archipelagos of rubble. We have a real thing for rubble these days, almost a philosophy of rubble. We understand that you should never completely atomize the last thing you built. Instead you should leave tantalizing hints of it in the storage box for the next time.

Spars of old staircases; doors and windows bodged together in promisingly unpromising ways. Every disaster contains a glimpse of the thing that will follow it.

It helps that even now neither of us is ever trying to build anything specific in the first place. Our cities belong to some doodling realm that exists in the margins, beyond the concerns of form and function. My daughter and I have an established interest in fantasy buildings, in unreal estate, and in the lives of strange, quiet people who are only an inch or so high. And I have come to see that all the places we build are, in some way, the same unmappable place, regardless of what shape they might take from one minute to the next.

Privately, I call this place the Inland Empire, a name I stole from the sand-blasted territory, just outside Los Angeles, where I was born. The Inland Empire! That term always seemed incongruously lofty when applied to a dusty collection of ragged-edge suburbs and sun-worn mini-malls done up in the Spanish style. It has the arresting quality of a printing error when you see it on the maps, too sweeping and romantic for a mere bureaucratic grouping of area codes, a constellation of drive-through Dunkin' Donuts. So I have rescued it and re-applied it. It fits much better with this shadowy, shifting space of our own devising.

And there are two tales to this city. The first is Leon's, of course. The lurching advances in building complexity match the explosion in her cognitive abilities as one idea connects with another, as plans form; as capabilities are discovered, as the images in her head have edged towards conscious thought. The first time we played, she gawped at the colours and shapes. Now, she stands bent over a box of bricks, searching through them for the single piece she is after. If it eludes her, she gets furious. When she finds it, she can ponder its optimal placement for the best part of a minute.

Then there's my story. For the first few months of our Saturday ritual, I now realize that I was witnessing something happening inside me. My fingers were growing numb, my limbs were getting heavier, I was becoming clumsier than usual. I picked up a slight quaver in my voice and injured myself in many small, stupid ways throughout the course of an ordinary day.

And then, at night, I would sometimes lie back in bed and discover that my mind was suspiciously quiet. There was not a single thought strolling around inside my head. It was an ominous kind of calm.

Over time, these early symptoms would reveal themselves for what they were. They were the first signs of multiple sclerosis, a maddeningly unpredictable neurological disease that I would spend the next few years trying, and often failing, to get an understanding of.

But let the night retreat for a few moments longer. I am grateful to Leon for all the time I get to build Lego with her. For the obvious reasons, and for this secret reason too: without Leon, I know that I would always build the same kind of structure – a low, rambling sort of building, something a talentless Frank Lloyd Wright acolyte might bang out for an inattentive client.

Together, though, Leon and I build all sorts of things. She cannot settle, and she rarely plans. She is always changing her mind, expanding her focus. The buildings she creates are daringly lopsided, or exist as bursts of freakish minimalism. A brick here, another balanced over there, and then: *done*. The purpose of these structures can shift very suddenly in the construction. A park becomes a prison when she adds a barred gate and then bricks in the see-saw. A skyscraper of mine can be utterly transformed by placing a single brick on top of it – she whacks on a ship's wheel and it's a galleon, set teetering through the seas.

This is the way she is with everything, going through that frantic period children have between two and four when everything is new, everything is possible, when everything is unprecedented and there is suddenly a real urgency to get it happening now, and all at once. I worry this will not last. I have seen the way older children play with Lego, when their parents visit us and the Lego is hauled out to entertain them. They make very pretty things, older kids, but it is a stale kind of prettiness. It is in debt to symmetry, in debt to the architecture of pedantry. It's a reminder of that thing Tom Wolfe said, that the middle years of childhood are the most formal years of your entire life.

And then one day you're my age and, when faced with Lego, you behave as I do. No rocket ships or alien worlds any more. Just pastiche, just real estate.

This is one of a million reasons why I need Leon. It is pure selfishness. She dreams of this stuff. And when she's awake, I now understand that she often thinks of it too.

And that worry of hers: *I see pictures in my head*, she explained to me through her tears, through her inability to land on the precise words. How did she know that? How did she know that the thoughts she was having were in her head?

What is multiple sclerosis? There are at least two answers to this question. The first is an attempt to explain the mechanism of the disease itself, a disease in which the body's own immune system decides to attack the fatty, insulating coating of the nerves in the brain and spinal cord. This coating, made of a substance called myelin, protects our nerves and speeds up those vital electrical pulses moving from one neuron to the next, kissing across synaptic gaps in a brisk burst of chemicals. Without myelin, crucial signals between the brain and the body become garbled or simply go missing entirely. The kisses go unmet, and over time you start to feel the consequences, in fingers, in toes, in glitch and twinge.

I envision the lightning-fast movement of these signals through my daughter as she learns to put nouns and verbs together for the first time, while I sometimes stumble over the simplest sentences. At times it seems that we are joined, the two of us, through the magical substance of myelin, as it advances through my daughter's brain and as it is attacked in my own.

Multiple sclerosis comes in a handful of different forms, depending on its severity. This book is concerned with relapsing-remitting MS. This is the most common form of the disease, in which new or worsening symptoms flare up in sudden attacks, or relapses, that can last anywhere from days to a few months before retreating. Over time, many people with relapsing-remitting MS go on to develop secondary-progressive MS, in which symptoms grow worse, with fewer periods of remission. In primary-progressive MS, the rarest and most aggressive form of the disease, symptoms grow steadily worse from the start, with no periods of remission. All forms of MS are powered by the same basic mechanism, however: it causes havoc wherever your nerves travel, and your nerves must travel everywhere.

This ties into the second answer: multiple sclerosis is a disease in which a diverse number of unpleasant things may or may not happen to you. It can affect almost every part of the body, causing anything from gently tingling fingers to full-blown paralysis, and in between you can get everything from incontinence to difficulty in swallowing, from fatigue to – in my case at least – bursts of euphoria. Multiple sclerosis can be life-shortening, but it is always life-altering.

Because of this, when someone first tells you that you have multiple sclerosis, it seems to me that they are not necessarily telling you very much. Over one hundred years after it was first described, much about MS remains mysterious. There are lots of blank spaces left on the map. Somewhere within these neurogenic wildlands lies the mechanism through which this disease springs its nasty tricks. Somewhere, most importantly for me, lurk the tricks themselves: all the bizarre and alarming and fascinating things that MS may do to you, which no one can predict.

My favourite description of MS is one of the very first: *marked enfeeblement*. That was the phrase the great French neurologist Jean-Martin Charcot used when lecturing the medical community in the late nineteenth century. Imperious and shy, a noble enigma, Charcot cared deeply for his patients, and yet he seems to have been able to view their suffering from a distinctly aristocratic distance. When he spoke of marked enfeeblement, he was referring to the various cognitive damages inflicted by a disease that he had been the first to accurately describe. Specifically, he was referring to MS's effects on memory, but he had time to address other problems too, such as the fact that new 'conceptions' are formed slowly in MS patients, and that 'the intellectual and emotional faculties are blunted in their totality'. I can attest to all this, and I should add a reminder that, even then, this is just the cognitive side of things.

If I was lecturing, as Charcot did every Friday and every Tuesday to audiences that often included many outside the medical profession, I would have to speak from muddy personal experience rather than academic curiosity, and I would argue that neurological diseases are ultimately an attack on individuality, in the same way that streptococcus, say, is an attack on the throat. Neurological diseases like MS live within the central nervous system after all, that complex tangle of 100 billion cells – every one a lightning bolt captured mid-strike – that makes each of us, through thinking, the person we *think* we are. When these diseases attack the brain, they cannot help but attack the person being endlessly remade within it.

It is perversely fitting that MS should attack the individual in such a fiercely individual manner. Every case of MS is different, and the sheer scope of the trouble it can cause is impossible to adequately capture. MS has a destination, and one I am all too aware of, but it has no set timetable, and it has posted no itinerary.

And at its worst, multiple sclerosis is nothing. A literal nothingness: the stillness of spasticity, the quiet of an addled mind. Day to day, I sometimes feel I am chasing a little pool of nothingness around inside me, the way I might tilt an air bubble up and down through a spirit level. Sometimes this nothingness seems to gather in the fingers, a lack of sensation that feels implausibly, paradoxically, raw. Sometimes it pools in the brain, a wordlessness, a theft of language that, on reflection, makes me wonder if I need nouns and verbs and adjectives in order to have any thoughts at all.

Since the beginning, I have always wanted to see this nothingness. I have not needed to understand it, perhaps, but I have needed it to take some kind of a shape before me. Early on it became clear what shape it would take too. Landscape has a way of creeping into language and filling it out. I talk of a chilly coastal fog that descends and swallows words and entire thoughts. I talk of the sudden erosion of context, as if a stretch of cliffside has been yanked away by a fierce tide. I talk of a *place* that I am transported to when the truly weird stuff starts to happen: my own Inland Empire. And it's not just the weird stuff any more. This landscape has become a way of thinking about what's going on with me day to day. It's a way of sounding out the boundaries of the world I now live in.

Perhaps the real change is in how I have come to see myself. I am a fretful man who has always dreamed of adventure. For thirty years I have doodled fantastical maps while talking on the phone or looking out of the window in class or at work; I have read books about experience while inching away from it whenever it seems to approach me in the real world. Now, experience is here and unavoidable: disease has forced me to become an explorer and a cartographer. Multiple sclerosis has ushered me into a new environment entirely, where the strange science of the brain intrudes into everyday life in unexpected ways and at unexpected times.

I'm not sure this perspective on disease is always the indulgence it appears to be. In the streets and intersections that Leon and I make of Lego, places that grow, contract and are endlessly being replaced, I get a fresh sense of the possibilities of space, of the ability of landscape to cope with change without any attendant need for understanding. You simply cannot get attached to what you have made when playing Lego with a child. You have to learn to deal with the sort of unpredictability that can pull up entire neighbourhoods with no warning, and that can then draw cathedrals out of the least-promising rubble.

And it's worth remembering that hidden within the diagnosis of multiple sclerosis is a second diagnosis: incurable. This is the one it can be truly mind-shredding to confront. Over the last three years I have come to comprehend what MS means on a day-to-day basis – the aches, the fatigue, the tingling moments when the whole world shifts briefly out of alignment – but it is much harder to understand that these things are going to continue, and only increase in regularity and force. Legs quake. Ribs creak. Sentences are cut short and plans are postponed as MS stages another guerrilla raid on context.

And so, in the months since my own diagnosis, my response has been to try to look outwards as well as inwards. My doctors have been working hard on me, establishing a treatment plan and plotting the likely course that this wilful, unpredictable disease is likely to take this time around. I have been busy too. I have had to find a new place for myself, and what follows is the story of my search.

This has been the objective, really, to get a sense of where illness has left me, to understand what this kind of illness – one that lurks inside the territory of identity – actually means for me. And perhaps what its various iniquities reveal about the mind I've been living in for the last thirty-eight years anyway – an idea of where the illness stops and I, often equally problematic, begin. I have seen so much, from the early sketches left by the first anatomists who sought to expose the godly architecture of the brain to the lunar world of today's MRI scans, silver and shimmering on computer screens. And I realize that over the last few years I've been slowly mapping my own body too. Alongside a growing familiarity with the buried treasures of the brain, I now know there are two nervous systems rather than one, for example, and I have a working understanding of the separate layers of the body's aggressive, and imperfect, immune defences. My search for understanding has brought internal spaces out into the light. It has stopped me from being quite such a tourist in my own skin.

This, then, is a book about my attempts to navigate the world as it appears to a neurological patient – a neurological patient who has just become a father. It's a book about trying to meet an unpredictable and inventive disease on its own terms. And it's a book about the brain, and about the things I have learned about the people who have struggled, over the centuries, to bring this strange, ugly, fascinating organ into the light and understand the way that disease affects it.

Because of all this, it's also a book about something that my daughter's Lego seemed to be stirring within me as we first got to know each other, an inkling, probably foolhardy, possibly obnoxious, that my diagnosis didn't have to be a total disaster, that its destructive nature might have some errant creative potential hiding within it. After all, there is only one rule when Leon and I build Lego: I must work with whatever she gives me. Even when she makes strange choices — such as deciding, halfway into a skyscraper, to stop adding new floors and turn the whole thing into a high-rise dog park — I must work with that and steer into it, rather than pretend it didn't happen or start again. Her gift is that she makes decisions I wouldn't think of, and so together we end up creating things that feel unprecedented to both of us.

I'm still doing all of that, I think, and it seems only right that Leon was there with me back at the start of all this. My daughter is my reason for exploring in the first place: I need to find a way to function as a parent with an encroaching disability.

People sometimes talk about how selfish having children is. They are talking, most often, about the planet, and they are reducing children to the barrels of oil they will consume, the plane seats they will fill, the beef or the quinoa that will have to be produced to feed them. I never argue with these people. Partly because I am timid, partly because I suspect they have a point, and partly because I have slowly come to recognize that having children is selfish in other ways too.

When I was young, twelve or thirteen, I had a very strong sense of what death would be like. Death would be like the evening of the last day of the summer holidays. Mawkishly you store your toys and you slump into bed. And then you lie in the warm, windless dark, staring at the ceiling or at the moon arcing slowly past an open window. And you think: I wasted all that. You think of the long summer days in which you got up late, in which you dawdled over breakfast, in which you could not make plans or decide, even, which direction to start out in for an aimless wander. You look back on this glittering opportunity and all you have is regrets at the things that didn't get done.

It never occurred to me that one day I might look back and feel that for every opportunity squandered there was one I decided to make the best of – or one, better yet, that I had no choice but to make the best of.

As I write this on a Thursday morning in the first half of 2017, I have just dropped Leon off at nursery. We rode the bus out there together – I'm sure we both chugged our way through some of the oil that should rightly belong to other people as we went – and she told me about Wonder Woman and Batman and a time, a few weeks ago, when she fell on the path outside our house and hurt her knee and felt, suddenly, that everything in the world was just terrible. Halfway through our journey, she zipped up her hoodie and then announced that she had forgotten what T-shirt she had decided to wear today and I had to try to describe it in great, forensic detail, the T-shirt under her hoodie, until she remembered that it was the one with the moose on it and that once she had put it on that morning she had had to take off her gold shoes and find a different pair because the gold shoes were just *too much* when combined with a moose.

We got off the bus and I explained, for the thousandth time, why she could not squirm out of holding my hand when traffic was nearby. We waited for the green man, we stopped in at the local Tesco to look at the new magazines, and she took the longest route to the magazine rack because, as she always does, she wanted to 'zigzag there and back'. We went to the nursery and found we were the first ones there today. She raced to a pole by the front door that holds up a small shingled roof, and she spun on the pole and then started to climb it. She tried to shout, 'Thunderbirds are GO!' but got confused, as she always does, and shouted, 'Ladybirds are GO!' instead.

She was too cool to let me kiss her goodbye when the doors to her nursery opened, or maybe she was still embarrassed about the ladybirds thing, so I waved her off from outside and got the bus home. As I creaked up the driveway a twinge in my upper leg announced that I was going to have to sit down for ten minutes fairly soon or I would pay for it later. I opened the front door on to the usual domestic crime scene: honey-flavoured hoops exploded underfoot, My Little Pony underpants flung over the arm of a chair, and toothpaste smeared across a cushion. Beneath the sofa, kicked there by a tiny foot, were the gold shoes that my daughter had decided were too much to wear that morning. I sat down and stared at them resting in the gloom there, and felt a wonderful, rich kind of sadness that the house was so empty.

And I realized once again: my world used to be vast, but now it is small and strange and bright, and I exist within it in a way I never did before. This is despite my current compromises. Maybe it is even because of them. My daughter sends me out into the world just as my illness is starting to shut that world down. Together we explore a landscape so compact that I can imagine a map of it fitting into the endpapers of a novel, but simultaneously so vivid and interesting that it belongs there.

The Marrow of the Skull

The birth of neurology and a basic guide to the brain

The study of the central nervous system began with a prod. Thousands of years ago, a man pushed his finger through a jagged hole that had been knocked in another man's skull in an accident, and pressed the soft matter inside to see if his patient would cry out and weep. Hopefully he would cry out: if the patient shuddered from the pain but did not vocalize his anguish, it meant that nothing could be done for him. Loss of speech indicated that a head injury was untreatable.

This was Egypt around 2600 BC, in the Third Dynasty of the Old Kingdom. And this was medicine as it existed at the strange, violent birth of neurology – not that it would be called that for many centuries. Doctors were priests in the Old Kingdom. Treatment sometimes involved crocodile excrement or prayer, or the milk of a woman who had birthed a son. And the brain was not the brain. Not quite. Not yet. Egyptians sometimes called it the marrow of the skull.

The phrase makes sense, I think. Without an understanding of the brain's centrality to mental life the skull becomes a bone like any other, and the thing inside it, though unusually grotesque and complex, might ultimately be no different from the paste and jelly found in any other bone. The marrow of the skull: here is the brain as an object. An object that we have struggled, over the millennia, to understand.

The Third Dynasty was a period of rapid cultural transformation for Egypt. Large-scale construction was sweeping across the empire, and turning Egypt into a veritable wonderland for head injuries as it went. Many of these industrial accidents were noted down in the earliest neurological writings yet discovered – a document known as the Edwin Smith Surgical Papyrus, which was not written by Edwin Smith (he was the archaeologist who purchased it in the 1860s) and which contains no notes on actual surgery.

This papyrus, which is sometimes said to carry the wisdom of Imhotep, the great priest and polymath, even though it was probably written a thousand years after his death, lists forty-eight medical cases and the best means of dealing with them. Twenty-seven of these cases are head injuries, and they offer a sometimes-confusing glimpse into the state of Egypt's thinking with regards to the brain.

Ancient Egyptians did not appear to value the marrow of the skull very much. The soul, they believed, resided in the heart. After death the brain was removed and tossed aside without ceremony during the burial process or, in the early days of embalming, simply left where it was.

Even so, the Egyptians clearly understood something of this strange, ugly organ. They noted that injuries to the head could cause dysfunction in distant limbs. They also recorded evidence that damage to one hemisphere of the brain would generally affect behaviour on the opposite side of the body.

Over the centuries, the brain's stature gradually improved. Today, we can marvel at the complexity and elegance of this compact bioelectrical masterpiece, even if many of our questions, such as how exactly do the brain's billions of electrical signals come together to create thought and consciousness, remain unanswered. We understand that the brain is where our sense of self resides. We have a growing appreciation of the brain's different structures. We have mapped a lot of the terrain.

My favourite map, although it is not unblemished by disagreement, is that of the triune brain, which was laid out in the 1960s by the neuroscientist Paul MacLean. MacLean argued that the arrangement of the various structures in the human brain tells the story of the evolution of the vertebrate brain in general – that it contains, in effect, three evolutionary strata. Most modern neurologists disagree with many of the details of his argument. Regardless, his three-part model of the brain remains a sprightly and easy-to-grasp outline of the brain's basic shape and function.

Working bottom to top, we move from the primitive territory of the brainstem, which controls the sorts of actions we have long since learned not to think about – breathing, the beating of the heart, bodily coordination – through to the limbic system, which is the territory of emotions and urges. The limbic system houses structures like the hippocampus, which plays a central role in the consolidation of memory; the amygdala, which is involved in the expression and production of fear and rage; and the thalamus, among other things the relay station that dispatches sensory and motor information out across the brain. The final part of the brain, resting above all this, is the neocortex – the rumpled cauliflower of conscious mind, each hemisphere split into four lobes that deal, between them, with everything from visual

perception and the comprehension of sound to concep-
tualizing, planning and logic. Breathing and laughter,
then fear and memory, and finally the human part –
mostly, it can sometimes seem, engaged in maintaining
the illusion that we are not entirely controlled by fear and
memory.

It can seem at times that this brain of ours is basically
a chemist, eager to whip up whatever magical cocktail
will keep you alive through the next five minutes of
unpredictable human experience. Your emotions are
frequently just chemicals – they're hormones, they're
neurotransmitters – and the brain dispenses them to
your body when it decides you need to feel their effects.
Over time, through exposure to this kind of thinking, I
have come to see the brain as a chirpy nineteenth-century
mixologist, with a starched collar and a centre parting,
knocking together fancy drinks and skimming them
down the bar towards me.

In my more melodramatic moments, I sometimes
worry about this mixologist, and what he might be doing
on the sly. The brain is very busy, and it does not show
its workings. It is looking out for you, but it is also operating without your conscious consent. It doses you with
oxytocin (playfully known as the hug hormone) to stop
you from skipping out on your family; it drops your consciousness entirely in times of danger so you can become
a creature of pure action and instinct. The brain and
conscious mind coexist, but the relationship is not always
fair. A brain hides things from you in order for you to
function. (I almost typed 'in order for you both to
function'.)

Putting the triune model to one side, the brain also
makes a kind of sense if you divide it down the middle,

into the left and right hemispheres. These two halves – endlessly invoked by expensive motivational speakers around the world seeking to explain the mystery of creativity – share a similar architecture, but evolution has equipped each to handle its own specialized functions.

And you could divide the brain in yet another way, carving it up between the grey matter and the white. The grey matter, composed of dendrites (the inputs of a neuron; the outputs are called axons) and cell bodies, is the part that has historically tended to get all the glory. Here, in the crackle of firing synapses, you get thought and action. The white matter, meanwhile, is often written off as mere insulation: a coating on the axons akin to the plastic flex you get on ordinary electrical cables. As we will see later, this perspective may be changing.

It is always interesting to know a bit of neuroanatomy, even at such a simplistic level as this. But it serves a deeper purpose for me. Imagine that the clumsiest cliché is correct and the brain really is just a computer. Then imagine that you open the computer's case one day and discover that there are termites inside who have been eating the plastic coating on all the wiring. What do you do?

2. Lost

The first time I saw my daughter, she didn't have a brain. A *neural tube* is the term I was given to help me process what exactly I was looking at. It was late December 2012, four days before Christmas, and on the screen in front of me, my daughter was a ribbon of plasticky flex, flapping at one end and knotted at the other. Not a heart, but the inklings of one. Not a spine, but the hint of the spine to come. Not a brain, not yet, but a brain would soon emerge from that knot, untangling neurons reaching out to form nerves that would connect the other parts of her together.

It seems odd even to use the word *her* in reference to that tube. She was not a daughter that day, but the most basic sketch of one — an outline, an ambition. Yet I loved what I saw on that hospital monitor. I looked at that flapping tube and thought: Yes. There she is. *Of course.*

Recognition. It had been a quiet night. Things to fix in the new house: cracked walls bubbled with old paint, winter winds treading slowly across the beams of the attic, the sound of dripping from somewhere dark and hollow and hard to pin down. Sarah emerged from the bathroom at around nine looking calm, and this immediately filled me with terror. Calm is the mask she presents to the world when the world itself is starting to shudder around her.

'I've had a bleed,' she said.

'Are you having the baby?' I asked too quickly, freshly stupid with the rush of panic. At six weeks, what I meant was: 'Are you losing the baby?' But I couldn't ask that aloud.

We used my phone. The helpline told us to go to the hospital the next morning. The night that followed was so long and restless that I refuse to remember it.

Instead, I remember the following day: the antenatal unit, cluttered with sagging Christmas ornaments, where we traded our identities for our medical circumstances. We were polycystic ovaries, and we joined the queue behind two IVFs and a third-trimester walk-in, feet spread, face not just damp but dripping with the effort of it all. There was no indignity to this new identity of ours, or if there was I didn't feel it – not that they were my ovaries. I simply appreciated the briskness with which the staff performed triage, cutting away our names to expose our needs, the way a paramedic might slice the clothes around a wound.

Tilt your head and she looked like a wound on the screen: a tiny dark tear in the pulsing, clotted grey fabric of Sarah's insides. They reach for the fruit and veg when a child is developing: this week they're the size of a bean, a fig, an orange. You can't help but feel yourself in the produce aisle, and you take some comfort in the mundane bustle of it all. But on the inside, they do not look like fruit or veg. They look like the secrets of life itself, the greatest of which is this: we are a central nervous system. That is the pared-back truth of us. The nervous system arrives first, and everything else is just collateral, the rusting gantry around an expensive rocket.

That heartbeat! That proto-heartbeat. The ragged, adorable fluttering of the neural tube that was now the bright point at the centre of our family. She seemed, what? Not determined. No, she seemed *assured*. She seemed confident. And maybe I could borrow some of that confidence – and return it later.

Coming home, blown about in the bus as it tackled the coast road just outside Brighton, Sarah put a hand on my face and told me: 'You were so calm.'

'I can handle the big things,' I said. She nodded. She knew. We both knew that the things I couldn't handle were the little things.

There is a story I often tell people about how my parents got together. I tell it even though nobody ever asks, and even though I have to then follow it up with the news that, by this point, my parents have been divorced far longer than they were ever a couple.

My parents got together in 1969. My dad was a silent-order monk from southern California, hitch-hiking his way around Europe in the middle of a crisis of faith. For most of the 1960s he had not spoken or even looked out of the window: his job as a monk was to pray for the world while remaining utterly removed from it. He had not heard popular music since the tail end of the previous decade, until one day a visiting Franciscan smuggled *Sgt. Pepper's* into the monastery so my dad could listen to it. He set it going on a record player rigged up in a Divco delivery truck he was meant to be restoring, and suddenly the monastery seemed far too small, and the world seemed like a thing that could not be saved from a careful distance.

My mum, meanwhile, was the teenage mod in the Hillman Imp who picked him up not far from Canterbury on a rainy afternoon. Three weeks later they were married, just days before Neil Armstrong walked on the moon.

All of us, I think, all of my brothers and sisters, feel a quiet kind of shame about the prosaic ways we met the people we fell in love with. I met Sarah in an office in Brighton. No hitch-hiking, no chance transatlantic encounters, nobody walking on the moon. I was temping between writing jobs, and she was the single glimpse of calm and competence and wit and warmth in a vast room filled with undertrained people, each of whom appeared to be seconds away from a calamitous error of some kind.

In deference to my parents, at least we moved fast. We got
together and then we got married, all within the space of a
year. Neither of us had seriously contemplated marriage before.
Neither of us really believed in marriage. And yet it was suddenly what we wanted to do. We got married before we even
lived together. At the back of my mind, maybe, there was a
slight anxiety: we had met in a rush, Sarah and I, instantly,
frighteningly in love from the start. In my experience, this
kind of love is almost always unstable. This kind of love cannot last.

I had not counted on Sarah's input, though. The stability we
needed came from her, this dark-haired, dark-eyed girl who
walked with her head thrust forward as if battling incessant
winds, and who frowned her way through conversations,
shuffling in the occasional crooked smile and a hint of that gor-
geously wonky incisor of hers, piecing each thought together
in the moment.

Before the office job, she had been a nurse, a witness to the
body's hidden mysteries. She had sutured wounds, knocked
back energy drinks in A & E, and had stuffed corpses with cotton wool – once a sister had opened a nearby window so the
soul could fly away, naturally. She had tended a giant skinhead
with a swastika tattoo who, coming around from the anaes-
thetic, panicked sweetly about the oven he was sure he had left
on at home. She had once stood on a chair in an operating theatre so she could look over the surgeon's head and see into the
cavity of another human being to watch the heart wriggling
like a bag of worms. Live bait.

'What was surgery like?' I once asked, and sensed immediately that I could not be told. Instead, she described how tired
she was when she went home afterwards. 'The fumes,' she said.
'In theatre weeks I was drugged out of my mind. The surgeons
get used to it.'

Nowadays she worked in health insurance, a job that relied upon her medical knowledge and her love of detail. By contrast, I wrote about video games. I have written about games for ten years and I tell myself that I have stuck with it because, beneath the flim-flam, the job is delicate and interesting. Games are perfect adventures for the timid but curious: bottle worlds where you can experiment endlessly with risk and failure. They also appeal because they seem singularly difficult to talk about. Writing about games involves trying to find words for things that are pretty much made to evade words. It involves diving beneath a game's surface fiction, and beneath its rules and restrictions and mechanics, until you reach the dim, muddy territory where the effects of all these things come together in the player's imagination. Down there in the ooze, writing about games has always seemed to me a bit like dredging an old river with a rich history of scuttlings and sinkings. That's the job, and I would give myself, in the grim shorthand of the review, a four out of ten. That is to say: noble intentions, but it didn't really come together, did it?

It came together in some ways, though. After a long period as a freelancer, I joined the editorial team of a website in Brighton shortly after Sarah and I got married. After years of floating about and nurturing a growing anxiety over the state of the freelance world, I suddenly had a bit of security. I had an office in town I could go to if I wanted, and a computer in the corner at home that I could work from if I didn't fancy the fifteen-minute walk in the morning. As I nosed slowly through my early thirties, I sometimes wondered if I should feel ashamed or deeply lucky that I had managed to preserve something that felt like a student lifestyle. I chose to feel lucky.

So we worked, Sarah and I, living lives that we decided were filled with incident although we rarely left the tangle of central Brighton. If there was a problem, it was one of emerging roles, emerging rituals. I was always worrying, and she was always talking me back to a place of safety.

She had training in this regard. Sarah has a hundred stories about her days working as a nurse. There are funny stories and shocking stories, but underneath these distinctions they are all compassionate and sad and filled with human understanding.

I often think of one story in particular. Long before I met her, Sarah spent six weeks as an intern at the Elderly Medical ward of the Royal Sussex County Hospital, a long room with the beds down one side, facing high windows and a speckled view of the grey Brighton seafront. Every morning she would rouse the patients from their muttering sleep and get them into their chairs ready for a cup of tea.

Dementia was always hovering, playful and vindictive. As Sarah moved down the line of beds, somebody would inevitably conclude that the thin room with the comfortable seats was the carriage of an old locomotive, chuffing through the countryside, probably during wartime and bound for somewhere exciting. The idea would spread, quickly and with little prompting. As she passed back along the line with the tea urn, she would ask everyone what they wanted for breakfast, and she would gently inform them, one after another, that they were not on a train.

As for me, I was always boarding some imaginary train or another, being whisked away in the wrong carriage, bound, it seemed, for a destination I had not chosen. I was always lost, often aggressively, fearfully lost. Eventually, even Sarah's brilliance at reorienting me started to make me worry. I worried that I was turning Sarah into my own personal nurse – and it was a kind of nursing that generated no entertaining stories of any kind to enjoy afterwards. What I fell for was her independence, that sense of a private life lived in a private world. Could I intrude on that without damaging it?

Still we rushed on. We talked of children, so we would need a house, and the one we were renting between us, which seemed to be almost all staircase, would not do. We saved and we borrowed. The house we eventually bought was a classic example of the easy kind of mistake we were always making. Sarah and I were both late to adulthood, and so we were always running to catch up. We raced into house-hunting, and that swiftly turned into house-buying, because we had found a place and instantly fallen for it.

Sarah liked it even before we set foot inside. She perched on the low fence that ran around the wildflower garden at the centre of the green that our estate agent had directed us to and breathed deeply. We had ridden the bus for twenty minutes – as far from Brighton itself as we would ever choose to live – and now we were in Saltdean, a secluded art deco suburb built around a concentric set of gently arcing streets. It was bright and cold, a lively July morning, with a playful wind to shuffle the leaves and carry the sound of country and western music drifting from the radio of a distant neighbour. The unfinished road around the green, lumpy and missing its coating of tarmac, was littered with chunks of rock that felt good beneath my shoes. The whole place seemed unfinished really, more like backwater America than subdivided East Sussex. It felt speculative, and it made us feel speculative.

Sarah was in a Huck Finn kind of mood from the start. She plucked a straw from the wild garden and started to chew. I knew she was making up her mind: *I love it*. We went inside: small rooms, but all of them filled with sunlight. Lots of windows, and not a straight line in the whole place.

The survey, when it came back to us, contained a litany of minor to middling structural offences. The detailing inside suggested a previous owner whose enthusiasm for DIY was only infrequently matched by competence. The house was extremely cheap for its location, and this was maybe down to the way the plug sockets were each settled at distinct heights in the walls, like birds finding their own perches in an old tree. It was maybe down to the way the radiators leaned out on rusted, cobbled-together legs of pipework, as if they were preparing to stagger across the room in the manner of the spindly alien tripods from *The War of the Worlds*.

None of this mattered, neither did the spreading mould nor the fact that the house had been on the market for the best part of a year with no takers. That actually helped bring the price even closer to our feeble range. The estate agent could have warned us of radiation leaks or curses from a wrathful pharaoh and it wouldn't have mattered.

If Sarah had given into an irrational love, I was not entirely innocent. In its layout, the house told a busy kind of story, starting as a two-room holiday cottage in the 1930s before growing, a room a decade, sometimes more, to form a surprisingly extravagant sprawl for a bungalow. The living room was at the centre now, and all the other rooms came off it – no corridors in the whole place. As a result, that living room had nine doors, and that reminded me of a story by Herman Melville, in which the narrator lives in a house built clumsily around an old chimney, with the result that his home is a muddle of converging interiors.

Should you buy a house because of Herman Melville? I asked myself the question and I heard the reply: Yes. Besides, all those rooms, those motley doors, had reminded me of something else too. Something a university friend had once told me many years back when we were lounging in the bar, caught in the busy period between failing to hand in one paper and failing to hand in the next.

His name was Matt, and at the time he seemed to be the wisest person I had ever met. In the bar that day, he said: 'When I've lived enough of my life to have achieved my ambitions –'

'Or,' I added, eager to appear fatalistic, 'to have seen those ambitions rendered impossible?'

'When I've reached that point,' he said, 'I'm going to buy a massive house, and I'm going to live inside it with a tiger. I'm going to just release the tiger into the house.'

'And then?' I asked. You always had to work at it with Matt.

'And then we're going to live entirely independent lives,' he said. 'The tiger and me. And each day will be a bonus day, a day that I will treasure, because I'll wake up knowing that one morning or afternoon soon, fate will bring me together with the tiger in the same room at the same time.'

'This is going to have to be a big house,' I said. And Matt nodded.

That had stayed with me: life with a tiger as a way to keep yourself in the moment. And occasionally life did feel like that. It felt as if you were being stalked, for your own good, by something wild and honest and far beyond the realm of nego-tiation. On the day we moved into the house, Sarah told me, amid boxes and bags and upended chairs, that she was preg-nant. She was pregnant. I could handle that quite nicely. I can always handle the big things.

But a house, I was about to find out, is not a big thing. It is a teetering stack of the littlest things imaginable, all of which are eager to fragment and require the involvement of specialized repairmen. Panic started to rise. Maybe a baby was not a big thing either.

We bought that house in July, when it was filled with light and the sweet domestic cooing of distant wood pigeons. When we moved in, however, it was December. Short days and dark. A fog had settled around the garden, the white walls of the liv-ing room seemed clammy and grey, and we were woken each morning by alien moans that turned out to be sheep on a nearby hill. Do you even let sheep out in winter? Somebody clearly did.

I sensed now that there were things wrong with this house, things that estate agents had concealed, that nobody else had spotted. Things that only I could see. It was wrong that the guttering was so bowed in front of the kitchen window, so clodded with moss, that it didn't collect the rain so much as curate it, turning it into a sad Vegas waterfall. It was wrong that shiny black insects would find their way into the strangest places, and that the cats didn't want to eat them – perhaps because they did not possess the elevated flavour profiles the cats had detected in the insoles of my shoes. It was surely wrong that the pipes in the house had their own bronchial voices, and that they would wheeze and cough all night, a wretched choir tuning up, as I lay fretting about the money it would cost to replace them. A typical story of my early interaction with the house runs like this: one afternoon, rooting around in the attic, I found a walled-off area with a hatch that, once I closed it, turned out to have no handle for opening it again – and a warning note scribbled on the front saying *Do Not Close*.

That winter, we painted the living room a seaside blue, and the nursery a lurid coral, but still: the house was making me spiky with worry. The whole thing. The entire potential expense of home ownership. A bullying kind of threat I could only counteract by carving my life into maxims.

'Most of the things you should worry about come down to water,' I told Sarah one day, apropos of nothing – maybe a leak beneath the sink, maybe a documentary about the Dambusters I had caught on TV. I was constructing rules and paradigms of fretfulness. The house had become a machine designed to make me unbearable.

'Do you know about this idea of being relatable?' countered my pregnant wife, who, at the time, was standing on a coffee table with a paintbrush, trying to reach a distant corner of the ceiling, while I was collapsed on the sofa, an arm flung over my face, deep into an impromptu therapy session. 'It's nearly un-imaginable that we can afford a house. Most people alive today can't. Many of your colleagues at work can't afford a house through no fault of their own, and our children will only dream of this sort of thing,' she said. 'This response of yours to extreme good fortune is not relatable.'

I knew she was right. Even so, I could not be shamed or shaken out of it. I gave up on any of the increasingly rare travel opportunities at work, and I often skipped the bus to the office and wrote at the desk set up in the spare bedroom instead. My wife was pregnant and my house was sick, infected with beetles and woodlice and rejecting all manner of expensive grafts. I felt I should stay at home with my patient. Not that it needed me. I clearly needed it.

And throughout everything, I had neglected to tell my own family we had moved. I have a big family. I am the middle child of five, which means that we all have to work up an aston-ishing amount of energy to impart news of any kind to one another. But my brothers and sisters deserved cards, at least, and my mother probably required a phone call.

And what about Dad? I kept thinking of a picture I had of my dad, standing, in the late 1970s, in front of the house we had owned in the redwoods of northern California. A huge timber place set back from a banked mountain road, a house that looms over him in the photo, casting a long shadow through the age-less trees. I could almost hear it creaking, that house, and when I looked at my dad he seemed so small against that massive frame, that encroaching forest.

Here, I told myself, is a man who would understand. Here is a man who would understand the insane, impossible pressures of owning a modest three-bedroom suburban bungalow on the south coast of England.

★

In terms of impending fatherhood, I at least did not feel the pressure of my lineage. My parents had blazed a trail that, even if it had been appealing to me, would be hard to follow. They are vivid people, my parents, both room-fillers in their own way. My dad was a social worker when we were growing up, and, although he never really talked about it, we knew what his job meant: it meant he went to work each day and saved children. A vivid career, and he was often vividly absent because of the hours he worked. I wince at a memory in which he returned home one evening and said he wanted to wash his hands. I led him upstairs, worried that he might not know where the bathroom was in his own house.

And when he was present, he was still vivid: the only American, seemingly, in all of Kent, his voice loud and genial in a world of sour muttering. It was an early indicator that if I was to earn the Americanness my passport bestowed upon me, I would have to work at it. Americans in the 1980s, which in provincial England were still so close to the 1950s, seemed to exude more colour than everyone else. My dad was a light source, even before he said anything, and when he did say something he was gentle and caring and somehow out of reach despite the smile. He was Harrison Ford with jowls and sad, watchful eyes, both inherited from his own father, who was a tyrant.

My mum was a different kind of vivid, prone to withering furies and fierce joy, forever in search of a cause, and forever finding one. She has only started to seem small in her sixties, when some of her internal furnaces have dimmed to soot and ember. She was unpredictable and often unfathomable when we were kids, and my sister and I agreed that we couldn't even be sure where she came from. Her family was French, allegedly: dainty surnames like Tuileries and Solei blunted by hillbilly Kent into Tilly and Solly. She looked like the product of a hundred different backgrounds, however: Romany in her dark-skinned sinew, mad-haired New York folk poet, strident babushka.

Together, Mum and Dad made strange, unintelligible life decisions, lurching back and forth between the US and the UK until everyone was dizzy. Like many people of that generation, the 1950s kids let loose in the '60s and '70s, they often seemed to conduct their lives as if they were governed by a regular casting of the I Ching. As a result, my early memories remind me of those View-Master machines that stored their 3D wonders on white cardboard discs studded with little slides: a bizarre assortment of places and sights, experience in search of a theme. That redwood forest, Mum spinning the car out on a curving mountain road when she turned a corner too fearlessly and saw a deer standing and chewing on the tarmac; a trip to buy a pumpkin in the countryside, sitting on Dad's itchy tartan coat in the back seat; the freeway at night, jumbo jets impossibly bright and still in the sky above Los Angeles. And then Kent, Mum's parents small, prim, and fanatics for a local variety of Christianity, all of us sleeping on the floor because a house of our own was only at the discussion stage.

Amazingly, these people had five children together. I was wedged between two older brothers and two younger sisters. I sensed that we had all been brought up without a great deal of forethought or planning, and I assumed that this cheery chaos was something I would bring to my own family, that it was in the genes on both sides. But I was not correct about this. My mum and dad had led a crazy life together when we were young, but the thrilling instability of their existence was a result of their relationship with each other. They were like two chemicals that erupted in combination but were quiet and safe when stored by themselves. When my parents separated, their individual personalities were suddenly visible. Dad, who eventually settled in Wiltshire, became shrewd and prudent, a planner and scholar of past experience. Mum, who stayed in Kent even though she hated it, continued to live like a house cat, somewhat tame, somewhat wild.

Which way did I lean? After a childhood with so little structure, the house I'd bought had kindled a new kind of panic inside me: responsibility.

And so I brought it with me, panic, to the twelve-week scan in February 2013, ready to argue that, this time, surely, it was at least an appropriate response. It struck me, at the time, as being surprisingly medical, this scan – short on the dreaminess and idle speculation I had been hoping for, nothing like my unhurried moments watching the gentle flutter of the neural tube.

The tube was gone now, replaced with a mass of early baby. Folds were measured, features were checked off and limbs counted. No time to stare into the screen and ponder what was taking shape; instead we were lurched from one thing to the next, Sarah and I somehow separated in that room by the force of our shared anxiety. We both experienced that scan by ourselves, and I alone remember a brief nightmarish cross-section in which the ribcage of my daughter suddenly loomed up through the grey bubble of her torso, looking like the mad splayed teeth of an anglerfish.

I sensed the mystery of the unborn child at that point. They are fragile, but they are terrifyingly powerful.

As we headed towards the twenty-week scan at the end of March, something started to change within me. Something that is apparent only in retrospect, in the same way that, when you find yourself lost on a journey, you must try to pace backwards to discover the moment you first started to drift.

The change was this: with no warning, and no obvious cause, my panic started to leave me. The house and its problems could not jolt me back to sparking life any more. I was serene, but it felt forced, like something that had been inflicted on me, as if a drum had been placed over my head to shield me from the world – and to shield the world from me. Was this the first sign of neurological problems? I am still not certain. It was remarkable, though. People remarked upon it. Sarah would say 'You must be feeling better' when a setback or a surprise failed to trigger a meltdown. I would nod politely and think: I'm not sure I exactly feel *better*.

There were still moments of lurid shock. My daughter was, at this point, a roving lump – an elbow, a knee, a fist – racing around under the surface of my wife's belly. At times, that lump seemed angry, but maybe it was just impatient.

And there was giddiness too. She loved buses, according to her excited wriggling, and she loved sugar and cold drinks and a TV advert that featured the song 'Moon River'. We told ourselves that we understood this girl who had yet to be born. We told ourselves that we would recognize her when she emerged.

By the twenty-week scan I was calmer than I had been for some time, and I assumed that this was a good thing. This final scan was serenity itself: a mild March day, a cheery sonographer, a wakeful baby who was gulping away with a mouth that looked just like my sister's. We moved in close and I saw the face of the full moon on the screen. Actually, I saw it twice: the left hemisphere of her brain, and then the right, creamy light riddled with pits of rich shadow.

And I was delighted by that illicit glimpse of such intimate territory, a vision of something that should generally go unseen. It was nice to feel calm, to feel no panic.

Throughout all of this, of course, there was one thing that should have caused me genuine panic. I missed it completely.

Illness is a perverse adventure. In its early stages, it runs you backwards, from experience to a clumsy sort of innocence. You unlearn things. You discover that old truths no longer hold. To put it more directly, one day you can open a door without incident. The next day you cannot. And yet you might not notice this change. Not for quite a while.

There must have been a first time, but I can't remember it. Without knowing it, I developed a full-blown problem with door handles. I started reaching for them and missing. One door and then another, a clawed swipe through empty air. Always a modest revelation, and this is because I never watched my hand as I reached for a door handle. I just assumed I would hit the target blind. After all, I always had. And then I would have to look and see that I had not hit the target.

It is a mildly amusing thing, to find yourself standing, hand extended and closed around nothing while the door you're trying to open just hangs there and remains shut. I doubt I gave it much more thought than that the first time it happened. Once I got the door open on my second attempt, I must have quickly filed the memory away alongside all other mildly amusing things, which is to say I forgot about it completely.

I also neglected to look for patterns, for waves rippling outwards from that first missed door handle, cresting gently over the other doors, the light switches, the kitchen cabinets and cashpoint keypads. For at least a year, or so it seems in retrospect, I failed to spot a silent disaster unfolding, a fundamental shift as the entire world and everything in it moved two or three centimetres away from me – but only if I wasn't looking.

It was hard to notice this when a baby was on the way, of course. As the due date approached, I fumbled through one day and the next, dropping things, spilling things, spiking myself on pen points and cutlery. I probably thought it was the anxiety of parenthood if I thought about it at all, and I didn't reflect on the fact that, actually, my anxiety had mysteriously vanished by this point.

So although I had told myself that I would recognize my daughter when she was born, that I would know her instantly and innately, this was probably unlikely. I did not know myself even. My hands had gone missing and I hadn't really recognized *that*. Sure, they seemed to be right there, snugly attached to the ends of my wrists. But when I used them for anything, they were often not quite where they told me they were. For the first time ever I began to have to look carefully at the distinct pieces of the world around me if I wanted to do anything. Pieces like keys and locks. I'd really look at them, I'd stare, because they had ceased to be objects of second nature to me. They had stubbornly made themselves visible through my growing clumsiness.

And still I couldn't take any of this seriously enough to wonder what it might mean.

You lose touch with yourself. Of course you do. The marriage. The house. The baby. Steadily, I found myself drawn back to my dad, often phoning him in the evening when Sarah had gone to bed, just to ask for reassurance: the Californian voice on the end of the line, the American talking to his English son. I remember listening to the phone ring, staring into the darkened window of our box room while I waited for him to pick up. I did this every other night. I even remember what I was generally thinking at these moments, the questions that prompted the call but would remain unanswered because unasked. *Can we do this? Are we allowed to do this?* I imagine that's what everyone asks themselves, and besides, I was surrounded by packing boxes, still unopened, of board games and video games and ancient copies of some of the books I had read and reread as a child and had never been able to throw out, all of which seemed to speak eloquently and rather damningly of my lack of ability to transition into the role of a parent.

What I don't remember is what I saw in that darkened

window on those nights. I was so used to my own reflection —
like I had previously been so used to door handles — that I never
really looked any more. My reflection was just an idiotic ghost
that followed me around in mockery, wild hair and wild beard
colluding with old brown clothes and a permanently distracted look to create the kind of person you might see in a
Depression-era photograph, huddled next to a dustbin that
someone, in a burst of community spirit, had set on fire.

Permanently distracted. But distracted by what? By my mid
thirties, the things I paid attention to were seismic, the sorts of
big-life things I would phone my dad about. My reflection?
Unlikely. And my door-handle problem? No chance.

A delivery room is no place for a baby: the submarine instru-
mentation, the echoing screams, the experts hovering with the
resuscitation trolley. Luckily, on a sweltering night in late
August, it's a monster who shows up: a sweet, scarlet Godzilla,
skin flushed and glossy and distinctly amphibian, eyes bright
and black, a fleshy beak for a mouth. Her head is lengthened by
the suction that has been applied to pull her out and as I lunge
for her while she's laid on Sarah's sweating belly, my first
thought is: I do not know this person, but she is a marvel.

'How is she?' cries Sarah. I stare in awe at my daughter's
head. Her black eyes stare back at me, perhaps trying to focus
for the first time. I try to connect the thin red face in front of
me with the baby who likes buses, sugar and 'Moon River'.
Her eyebrows are two faint lines, as if drawn on with pencil.
She seems to be pondering something difficult. She seems to be
very old. She waves me aside.

'How is she?' cries Sarah again, and I realize I didn't answer
her the first time. I realize that some foolish part of me has been
waiting for my daughter to speak.

A day later, we wrap her in blankets, cardigans and scarves, even though it is late summer, and lock her into her car seat to take her home. My dad drives us away from the hospital. We are still wordless with emotion. I probably fumble with the door when getting her out of Dad's car. I probably reach for the handle and miss. I am still waiting for the moment of recognition with my daughter.

And then it's there. The next morning I wake up with my hand up against my eye, and my daughter, lying just beyond me, looks truly tiny in comparison. This is not a trick of perspective, I discover: she really is that small. And when I pick her up, she is so implausibly light. She is pleasantly rigid, but as insubstantial as an egg carton. She wakes and stares at me, dark eyes canny and curious. Her mouth starts to work: she is gulping. I pass her, reluctantly, to Sarah, who has just emerged from a very thin sleep. My daughter keeps those dark, wet eyes on me for a second, or at least she seems to. It's enough. Something has passed between us. It feels like we have had our first moment together.

We spent the next few weeks staring into our daughter's face. I wasn't searching, I don't think, but I was still waiting for something, even if I didn't understand exactly what it was.

Maybe I was waiting for her to settle. She changed every day. Her eyes started to lighten to a marbly blue. Her cheeks grew dimples. She learned to smile, her first attempts followed immediately by a frown as she studied our reactions.

Between her transformations, Sarah and I assumed certain roles. Sarah was food and I was sleep. (Sarah was frequently sleep too; I was never food.) Leon woke very occasionally and, blearily examining us, either smiled or burst into tears. When there were tears I drove myself mad trying to stop them. Mix tapes were created of songs she had wriggled to in the womb, articles in progress were read to her in a slow, narcotic voice:

she was soothed by game reviews and developer interviews, by list features and picture captions. Everything worked at least once, but nothing worked for ever. We were always searching for ways to please her.

I remember a few things particularly fondly from this period. The first time I attempted a nappy change was a bit of a sitcom, if anybody ever made sitcoms about bomb disposal. 'I'm going in,' I said to Sarah, and then shut the door to the nursery behind me. Seconds later Sarah opened it, largely out of curiosity, and in those seconds Leon had managed to pee all over herself and me. Her hair was wet with it, which was quite a trick, and I appeared to be going into some kind of traumatic shock in the corner. Sarah moved me gently out of the way and became an A & E nurse again. 'Don't worry,' she said as she worked. 'This is not the first time I've been pissed on.' As my senses returned, I marvelled at what a fascinating person I had married.

Defeat like this was generally amusing with Leon. Days later, though, I had a crucial victory in the same nursery. I was changing her for bed and she started to sob. I watched her face contorting with sadness, little eyes reduced to pooling slits, little chin wobbling. I thought I was going to freeze again, but instead I realized that I knew exactly what to do. Nobody had ever told me, I just knew. I reached forward very gently and placed my hand, suddenly huge, on her tiny chest. It took a second to calm her completely, and then we stared at each other for several minutes, lost in sheer fascination.

The three of us went out together once during this period. Our mission was to get her registered at the local council, to announce to the world the name that we had spent weeks piecing together: Leontine Maple Donlan. I can't remember the trip at all. All I can remember is the preparation, the first time we needed to put Leon in anything more complex than a

vest that buttoned up at the bottom. We had great ambitions
for that day: a shirt, trousers, a jaunty bonnet. It was our first experience of clothing anyone other than ourselves, and it felt
like the moment in a Tintin book where the flustered kidnapper
has to bundle a chloroformed victim into street clothes before
they can be propped up in the passenger seat of a car.

Better to stay at home. Over the months that followed, even
after I returned to work, I chose to work from the spare room.
In the mornings, Leon would awake next to us, still impossibly
small and yawning. In the evening she would lie on me and I
would stroke her tiny spine, running a finger up and down its
ridges to soothe her while we watched documentaries about
Nazi megastructures and all the trouble that polar bears were
suddenly in.

The lunchtimes were the best times: she would sleep on the
bed, and Sarah would doze next to her between feeds. I would
come in from the spare room and lie there, looking out of the
window of our new house – so new still that the bright yellow
leaves of our neighbour's backyard tree still seemed thrillingly
exotic against the blue sky – and I would read and think about
my daughter growing up.

It was not idle reading. I worried about being a father. It suddenly seemed that the books I had been living with my whole life
were absolutely filled with them, fathers, and they were either
implausibly, unreachably life-enhancing or they were total disasters. The perfect dad is a cliché, and so is the brute, and there
seemed to be no middle ground at all.

Inevitably, I decided to use books to solve the problem that
books had created. I would fight books with more books, and
so I bought books on child development, books on child safety,
books about toddler diets and books about the importance of
pre-school education. If your child does not attend an enrich-
ing pre-school, these books informed me, they are likely to

become a monster. The soft skills will not develop. They will not connect with people. They will have no empathy. There are hundreds of books like this, all eager to pitch their own disasters, all filled with their own monsters.

And I had been buying other books too. Alongside the child psychologies and the conflicting instructions, I had been slowly collecting a selection of the books I had when I was young. A gift for my daughter, I told myself, even though I knew that it was more likely an indulgence for myself.

I read the *Spy's Guidebook*, a template for summer busyness with its matchboxes full of secret-agent trinkets, its codes to chalk on walls or scratch in the earth. No bullies in the *Spy's Guidebook*, just enemy spooks. I already worried about future bullies. Then I read Ellen Raskin, her mystery stories alive with puzzles and nominative determinism, with a hard-won mistrust of adults and the things they do to children – and to themselves.

Back when I first read them, these books all fed into my favourite childhood fantasy, which was simple, thrilling, and entirely useless as a preparation for meaningful adult exist-ence. My fantasy was that everything in my life was a clue, and only I could put them together. I felt this almost all the time as a kid, to varying degrees. Maybe everyone does. A gust of wind on leaving the house or the right strain of light slanting through branches overhead could trigger the sensation that I was entering a *moment* and must pay attention, must try to understand what was happening around me. I collected things I found: broken glass, scraps of paper with other people's half-finished notes. I drew maps, in which I kept track of the layered, often invisible, aspects of the environment I lived in, and I sensed a deep order in the world, albeit a hidden order. Even then I did not need to understand it. I just wanted to *see* it. I just wanted to explore it.

I did not assume that Leon would come to think these sorts of things too, but I did wonder what private interactions with the world she would choose to conduct. And I sensed that her arrival might require something new from me – or maybe even something old that I had almost forgotten.

I read on. Late summer became autumn, and then winter. Eventually, I washed up on *Treasure Island*. The best edition: the Everyman Library one, with the map at the front followed by illustrations from Mervyn Peake, who conjured grotesque pirates and set them playing among ferns and bracken. Peake draws sunlight by leaving it out: he draws around the light and then it just radiates off the page. He never draws Long John Silver the same way twice, and his old blind Pew is truly a monster, a thuggish lump with a howling gape of a mouth, hands grasping and their reach unthinkable.

I had always known that *Treasure Island* is a dark book, a book with a child's morality, but I had never seen that quite as clearly as I did with Leon lying next to me. Although she was rarely up for more than an hour or two, and she generally limited herself to thrashing her legs or smiling very specifically at things nobody else could see, she had somehow crept into the ageless text and rewritten sections, playing up the dangers, underlining the menace. Most of all, she had worked on the book's central moment. Young Hawkins, Jim lad, has taken to the sea in search of treasure. And now, hidden in the apple barrel in the galley of the *Hispaniola*, he is overhearing the details of a mutinous plot brewing among the ship's crew. This is all led by Long John Silver, whose murderous deceit is becoming apparent soon after Hawkins has started to see him as a friend, almost a parent. This is deception not just of the upper crew, then, but of a child who has grown to love him – who had assumed, in that childish way, that he was loveable.

For the first time ever, it was a relief to finish *Treasure Island*.

We had a quiet Christmas, just the three of us, and as New Year's approached, I picked up *Dr Jekyll and Mr Hyde*. More monsters of pragmatism. And at the start of *Hyde* there is a door. A door with something of a mystery to it.

One January morning in 2014, I lurched upright in bed at around six and announced: 'I think I'm having a heart attack.'

The main audience for this was Leon, five months old and sharing the bed with us, often sleeping sideways and leaving little snow angels in the sheets. On less catastrophic mornings, she would double as my alarm clock, a warm foot in the face telling me it was time to get moving. (I would often leap from bed to discover, in the chill air of winter in an old, rattly house, that this alarm clock was malfunctioning, and it was still before five.)

Next to her was Sarah, squashed up against the wooden bars of an open-sided cot that we'd clamped on to the bed. To accommodate the smallest person, who somehow required the most space, we would both end up sleeping in right angles, facing away from each other. Parenthood has a mysterious geometry all its own.

At the time it seemed that Leon was an amalgam of the two of us, that she fluctuated between resembling Sarah and resembling me. When she was storing up energy she ate and ate and her head changed shape. She became a moon-face like me: round and pale and wide, built for expressing wonder or confusion and little else. When she was growing, she reverted to Sarah as her skull seemed to lengthen. She shifted from Méliès to Modigliani: a blonde Modigliani, amused but otherwise unreadable.

Her temperament fluctuated too, but here she was firmly her own person – two of them, in fact. Watchful one second and endearingly dictatorial the next, both states were enlivened by an eagerness to break off from whatever she was doing and find something in the world that surprised her. Whatever shape her face took, her mouth was forever playing with the start of a smile. She even smiled before she burst into tears.

Wordless at five months, Leon was not fazed by my announcement that morning. Intrigued and amused, she sucked her thumb and considered me at length, waiting to see what happened next.

Sarah, more used to my cheery opening gambits, propped herself up on her elbows and squinted.

'Pain in your arm?' she asked.

'No.'

'Pain in your chest?'

'No.'

She flopped on to her back and blinked. 'What's happening exactly?'

'My hands feel too tight,' I said, as I placed my palms together and squeezed. I steepled the fingers and then pushed them against each other.

Nothing looked particularly swollen, but the flesh was prickly and hot, as if my skin were suddenly being forced to accommodate much larger bones. I sensed an imminent rupture, probably fatal: sausages splitting on a grill. 'It's like I'm toasted or vacuum-sealed or something.' I struggled for an adequate description. 'My hands feel like Pop-Tarts.'

Best to keep the sausages to myself.

'Your hands feel like Pop-Tarts.' Sarah rolled over. 'Doesn't sound like a heart attack,' she said as she closed her eyes. 'Sounds neurological. Much more likely to be multiple sclerosis or something.'

While Sarah slept, I went into the bathroom, taking Leon with me. Leaning her over one shoulder so I could feel her warm breath on my cheek, I pinched my fingers and felt pins and needles radiating outwards around my knuckles. My most reliable sense of identity has always resided in my hands, I think. In my mind's self-image I am still about sixteen, stumbling and elbowy inside a flapping shirt and billowing cord flares. My hands, though, speak to the person I would like to be today: precise and gentle.

But this morning I did not recognize my hands. They were filled with strange electricity, dangerous and uncontrolled, as if a sparking cable were jolting itself around inside me. I looked at my wedding ring, which has never really fitted properly and has worn a neat little groove where it rests. I tugged at the ring and gently eased it upwards. The groove didn't seem to cut any deeper, as I would have expected if my hands were truly as puffy as they now felt. The coloration of the skin didn't seem any angrier. Yet it was hard to say this with any certainty.

I realized that I was not prepared for illness, if this was illness. I had not taken stock. I did not know myself.

I propped Leon up so that she was sitting on the rim of the sink, leaning against me, and I placed my palms against the cold tiles beneath the window. The sparking in my hands didn't stop, but I could at least get a better shape of it here. It was not my entire hands that were electrified, just the fingers – just the very ends of the fingers in fact. Maybe I've slept funny, I thought, eyeing my daughter, who eyed me back. She wanted to see the wedding ring again, its gold catching the morning sun and igniting patches of the grey light of the bathroom.

Slowly, a memory of the day before returned to me. In the office, writing an interminable review about an interminable game. Dividing my time, as usual, between the keyboard and the control pad. Suddenly, my work seemed like so much abuse aimed at my hands, as if I were sending them down into a salt mine every day and expecting them to do all this mindless toil without complaining.

After work, I had gone out to dinner with a few friends – my first night out since Leon's birth – and I now remembered that, while I was fumbling around for a tip, I briefly felt something new happening in my fingertips. A sort of pinching effect, as if somebody had placed crocodile clips across the nails. I shook my hands a few times, and then made an easy peace with it when I noticed everyone had stopped to watch me. An occupational hazard: soldiers get shot, firemen get burned alive, and people who write about video games for a living get hunched backs and tingling fingers.

I was still staring at my hands when Sarah eventually came into the bathroom and started brushing her teeth. She had her phone with her, and the screen blinked and flashed with her latest craze: an app that allowed her to track vessels moving through the sea that lay less than a mile from our house. This had been her reaction to our new home, perched on the edge of the coast. As I ranted about bargeboards and soffits (without ever quite understanding what either of these actually is), as I filled myself with tedious knowledge, like the names of the curved tiles that run along the backbone of a roof – they're called bonnets – she had been drawn towards the sails and the silver horizon: yachts and fishing boats and huge shadowy tankers passing in the darkness.

'That Russian yacht is back,' Sarah said. 'The millionaire's one.' It was a favourite, a wallowing bleached thug that appeared by the marina every few months. And then she clocked my carefully prepared expression: noble suffering, revealing itself despite obvious stoicism. 'Still feel weird?' she asked. 'Maybe it's your version of the fireworks.'

This thought had occurred to me: that there was something of a reversal taking place. While fretting about illness is definitely my territory, Sarah's usually the one who wakes us all, a light but voluble sleeper, forever being ejected suddenly from some dream or another, babbling insanities. None of this is a criticism. If anything, this tendency of hers has meant that our relationship has always been peculiarly intimate. I know the sorts of things that happen when she closes her eyes.

And 'My hands feel like Pop-Tarts' could have been her line. Two nights before my fingers started tingling, she awoke me with frantic talk of fireworks erupting over water, colourful and bright. 'Did you see the lights?' she asked. 'Did you see the lights in the sea?'

'That's the subconscious,' I said at the time, and nodded to myself. 'My dad says that when you dream of the sea you're always dreaming about the subconscious.'

'Your dad says a lot of things,' said Sarah. The fireworks faded and the sea withdrew, but in the bathroom that morning my hands still felt weird.

Even so, there was little sense of genuine fear. I was still living with the volume down, everything that happened was just voices bleeding through from a distant room. Once we were all up, my fear of a heart attack faded, and so I was left to explain away my tingling hands in a less alarming manner, inattention giving ground to denial.

And the denial worked like this: didn't my hands often tingle a little these days? And if they did, when had that started? When had my back started aching, for that matter? When had my feet started feeling pinched and heavy? 'This isn't illness,' I told Sarah as I dressed Leon. 'It's so much more awful than that. It's old age.'

'It's middle age,' laughed Sarah. 'Doesn't that sound even worse?'

It wasn't middle age, but I'm not surprised by the category error. I have had to work at being ill. I understand that now. I have had to work at the interpretative side, the filing side, the side that covers the whole muddling business of learning to live with illness. It has been real work too. Grinding work. At times, it has even felt like physical work, in a dull kind of way, as if I have been polishing the lens of an old telescope so as to see distant things more clearly, more precisely.

And I understand that the nature of the work itself is always changing. For a year or more I missed a range of increasingly worrisome neurological symptoms because I did not know how to do the intimate work of discovery. Self-involved as I have always been, I did not yet know how to reach inwards, to feel out the hidden sensations of consciousness, to take a single cognitive oddity and look for the wider patterns it might fit into. (Later on I would encounter the opposite of this: I would grow so attuned to changes inside me that I would sometimes spot things that weren't there. I would invoke phantoms.)

With my tingling hands, the work was very different, however. I did not know how to tackle denial. I did not know how to dodge my own lies.

In truth, I was becoming increasingly electrical. Static was building up inside me, spreading out from the tips of my fingers and along my arms, spreading up from my toes and through the balls of my feet and into my legs. I was getting an origin story without the superpowers to make it worthwhile.

All of January, I told myself that nothing was happening, even though it clearly was. Instead I argued that the tingling could not last. It seemed such a small, insubstantial thing, even if it was steadily taking over. It was beginning to push me around too. At night, I could no longer do up the tiny buttons on Leon's bedclothes after her bath. In the morning, I often could not feel my fingers at all, just a fidgeting mass of pins and needles at the end of my wrists, and beneath the tingling there were rubbery hands, like a prop from a joke shop. But still, I managed to find excuses. I was sleeping funny, what with three people sharing a bed made for two. I had pulled something in my neck when I carried Leon in the sling. Fatherhood itself was undermining me even as it continued to delight. The first laugh. The first true look of recognition. The first moment I reached into the tumble dryer and an implausibly tiny pair of trousers came out along with the duvet cover and kitchen towels.

Then, in early February, I found something new. One Saturday I found myself asking: 'Do you ever get that thing? That thing when a motorbike rushes past outside, and it's so loud that you feel the sound in your spine?'

I phrased this question very carefully. I made it breezy – unnaturally breezy – because I had a vested interest in receiving a breezy answer in reply. Even as I spoke, though, I knew I was in trouble. Sarah's face started to sag as I reached the halfway mark. When a smile sags, you don't get a look of sadness. It's more a look of disgust that emerges. Accidental disgust. Disgust delivered in the place of fear, which is following behind it and needs time to catch up.

'No,' said Sarah eventually. 'Nobody ever gets that thing.'

We were in a coffee shop, and the fact is that a motorbike really had just rushed past. And it had been loud. And as it passed, I had involuntarily ducked my head and felt a revving explosion, a sympathetic chugging of wide-band electricity as it roared down my spine and into my limbs, finally free from whatever opposing forces had held it back.

I laughed stupidly: to buy time to think of something to say, perhaps, or maybe because I was stupid with surprise at what had happened. If that pulse of sheer energy hadn't come from outside, if I hadn't been rattled about by traffic, then I had just experienced the strangest thing to ever take place *inside* me. Something a thousand times more powerful than the tingling in the fingers. My tingling: tingling I suddenly realized I had come to accept as a part of me.

Slowly, I tilted my head again. Join me. Bring your head forward, so that your chin descends until it touches the very top of your chest. What do you feel? Nothing, I imagine. But there is a world of sensation you are missing out on: a gentle buzzing that starts as my head begins to move, and that suddenly catches, becoming a fierce corrugated shudder, broad and thick and somehow undeniably friendly, building at the top of my spine and then racing downwards, lighting up my innards as it goes. It used to burn itself out in my lower back; now it tends to turn to embers in my calves. Over time, I have learned I can control it a little: I can play it like a musical instrument, pausing my head at certain spots and lengthening the rumble that's produced, changing its shape and its complex, endlessly threaded patterns of energy.

I felt it a second time in the coffee shop. The rush of electricity, but with no motorbike to blame it on. 'Um,' I said, and then: 'I think this might be serious.'

'I know,' said Sarah. We got up to go, coffee half-finished. We both understood that I couldn't waste any more time than I already had.

Wasting time is relative, of course. When I look back on those early days, I realize that it is the privilege of an explorer to name the things they find. Some get to name places and creatures, strange rock formations and hidden bays. I get to name sensations. Generally, yes, these sensations have names of their own already, but I can make them mine with private terminology – and it is the private terminology that lasts.

In retrospect, those first three weeks of growing unease gave me so many new names to play with. Pop-Tarts: that's a name that's stuck. I still talk about Pop-Tarts when my hands feel tight on waking. I still talk about radio static in my feet and arms, and when it gets bad I tell my wife that I have been set to vibrate – a private vibration that only I can feel, spreading down my arms and my thighs, warm and annoying because it hides the buzz of my mobile phone when it alerts me to a call or reminds me to take a pill.

One thing I have never renamed, however, is that vast rush of energy down the spine. The medical name for it is Lhermitte's sign, and it is Lhermitte's sign I have chosen to stick with. It was not my first symptom, but it was the first that Sarah and I tracked down and looked up, the very first private incidence of neurological wildness that I was surprised to discover had already been mapped. 'An electrical sensation that runs down the back and into the limbs. In many patients, it is elicited by bending the head forward.'

Lhermitte's, I now understand, suggests a lesion, or scar, on the spinal cord. If I had ventured this far down the Wikipedia article I would have discovered that this, in turn, can be caused by a lot of things: enough at least to allow me a few more weeks of sweet denial before I saw a neurologist.

But denial suddenly wasn't so sweet any more. It had become flimsy. Partly because Lhermitte's was too bizarre and forceful an imposition ever to settle into a comfortable space in my life, and partly because of something I read when I first looked Lhermitte's up, a detail that seemed to speak with a worrying clarity about the world I was entering: the landscape of the central nervous system.

Lhermitte's sign, the passage explained, is not actually a sign, but a symptom, since a sign is objective evidence of a disease that should be apparent to everyone, but a symptom, like Lhermitte's, is subjective – a private madness that cannot truly be shared. Furthermore, the sensation was first described by neurologists Pierre Marie and Charles Chatelin in 1917; Jean Lhermitte, a neuropsychiatrist, only came to it three years later – and only properly wrote it up four years after that.

A tiny oddity, but still: Lhermitte's sign is not really Lhermitte's sign. Welcome to neurology.

The Man Who Couldn't Open a Door:
A guide to proprioception

Before I had my own neurologists, I had Oliver Sacks.

Sacks feels like the best kind of personal physician, his gentle voice speaking to you straight out of the page as he discusses the many cruel deficits that neurology trades in. My favourite of his books may look like collections of Sherlock Holmes stories – and the case histories they present have titles that any detective would be happy to have tidied away in the files: 'The Man Who Mistook His Wife for a Hat', 'The Visions of Hildegard' – but these mysteries are solved by kindness and quiet perception rather than violence and the clanging arrival of justice.

Over the years I would occasionally read that Sacks was not always considered to be a great clinician. Some have argued that he exploited his patients by turning them into literature. I found that last criticism false as soon as I became a neurology patient myself. Sacks gives the newly diagnosed permission to find their predicament interesting and human. He says: This is not the end of experience, but the beginning of a new strain of experience. He says: What is happening to you has value.

At times in the early months of my own neurological confusion, when I was fumbling with handles and light switches, I would imagine myself as a character in one of Sacks's narratives. 'The Man Who Couldn't Open a Door', perhaps, or 'The Case of the Misplaced Hands'. But what I did not realize was that Sacks had already tackled this problem I was having – albeit from a far more frightening vantage point. What does it mean to misplace your body? he asks in a story titled 'The Disembodied Lady'. It turns out that the stagy Wellsian nightmare conjured in that title is well earned. To misplace your body is the stuff of horror.

'The Disembodied Lady' describes an encounter between Sacks and a patient who has lost not just her hands but her entire physical being. Christine, a young computer programmer, is admitted to hospital to have her gall bladder removed. On her first night in the ward she dreams that she is losing control of her limbs, and when she awakes, the dream has come true. Over the course of a few days, simply standing up becomes impossible, while her hands start to wander by themselves if she isn't looking at them.

A complete disintegration of her body's awareness of its own spatial reality is under way. There is no cure. But with time, Christine is able to make a partial functional recovery through compensating systems. When Sacks leaves her at the end of the narrative, she is guiding each movement by sight – an exhausting, debilitating workaround. 'I feel my body is blind and deaf to itself,' Christine tells Sacks. 'It has no sense of itself.'

'The Disembodied Lady' exists within the strange spook country of proprioception, the means – along with vision and the balance organs of the vestibular system – by which the body creates a sense of itself in space. Proprioception is a deeply physical business, and yet it's simultaneously a largely intangible one. It is not just the brain's idea of where the body is from moment to moment. It is part of what makes a person's physical experiences feel real and personal in the first place.

This process depends upon sensory receptors called muscle spindles that are attached to individual muscles throughout the body, alongside the motor neurons. The motor neurons convey signals from the brain telling the muscles to move. The sensory neurons relay information about movements back to the brain, so that the brain can then construct an idea of exactly where everything is – a sense of what the hands are doing, where the feet are resting, whether the back is bent or straight, and even whether a person is speaking too loudly. A proprioceptive deficit is therefore an intelligence deficit: it means that the messages being sent back to the brain are not being properly understood.

Most people have little need or opportunity to acquaint themselves with proprioception, for the same reason you don't often ponder the dance of electrical energy and resistance that occurs when you fire up your kettle. Generally, this stuff just works. Proprioception is a guiding hand so deft and considerate that you might never come close to spotting it, and this is the tragedy of the body's most elegant systems. You only learn how clever they are when they break – and when it becomes a matter of how clever they once were. I feel lucky, in a chilly, rather blasphemous way, to have been given this fleeting glimpse of the inner workings, just as I feel lucky that proprioception was my introduction to the world of neurological disarray. I suspect that proprioception is an ideal introduction: a gentle indicator that there is always a level of mediation between the world and our experience of it.

As Sacks explains, however, a proprioceptive deficit isn't always so gentle. What has happened to me is nowhere near as all-consuming as what happened to

Christine. She had horror; I have had pratfalls. A very slight deficit has turned my house into a riot of impediments. My shins are constantly bruised from chair legs and low tables, while a cat becomes a silent-movie set-piece as it darts about, brushing in and out of flickering zones of awareness, sending me into an elbowy panic. I go to the kitchen before bed to get a glass of water, and my wife hears the enthusiastic Foley effects of a man klutzing through the darkness, even though all the lights are still on.

At its most insidious, though – and I wonder, honestly, if this is still neurological territory or something else – the comedy retreats a little. The mystery of proprioception seems tangled up with its mundanity. Over the last few years, my relationship with my own domestic landscape has become ever so slightly dreamlike: I'm left endlessly exploring places that I should already know – and making fresh discoveries. Light switches in my house fascinate me: I swear they take playful journeys up and down the walls, settling at unlikely heights.

I have read about this sort of thing too, but not in Oliver Sacks's books. Philip K. Dick was troubled by light switches moving around, never settling quite where he remembered them being before. He saw this as proof that the world was being edited and updated around him. I don't really blame him. How could I? It is a small step from neurological complaint to generalized ontological conspiracy.

Part of the reason I struggled to see the problems I was having with proprioception is that they seemed so personal, so private, so tightly woven into the texture of my life that I could not be sure they hadn't always been there. It is hard to spot the things that happen when your brain starts to go wrong, because your brain is the last thing that is going to be able to tell you about it.

Yet Sacks could tell me about it. And here is the thing I will never get used to about neurology: when you finally look up some private and wordless sensation, you often find that it has already been catalogued and codified. You discover that it is not as private as you have suspected, or as wordless as you have feared.

3. Help Me

I was twenty-five when I saw what the brain can do.

Dawn in a house that my brother and his wife had recently bought – tall and thin with a spine of creaking staircases running through the centre, surrounded by old rooms perfect for the clattering passage of young children, none of whom had yet been born. My dad had woken me from the sofa in the lounge. He took me up to the big bedroom on the first floor. Inside, my brother was having a grand mal seizure.

I did not want to see Ben having a fit. I had felt, up to this point, that I could either be stoical or informed, and I had chosen stoicism. Dad, however, seemed to understand that I was faking adulthood, that I was a large child loose in the world and that nothing real had ever happened to me. There are ways I have learned to avoid becoming an adult. I can't drive. I never organized a pension until the government did it for me.

I have avoided thinking about this moment for the last decade, and so the memory is bright and sharp and undisturbed. I almost feel like I could reach out with my hand and push through some invisible boundary, the air parting in thick, mineral clods, to find myself back in that room, a red shirt hanging over the mirror, water spilt from a glass and exploring the grooves and divots of the bare floorboards. Ben is laid out on the bed in the recovery position, and Dad stands over him. Ben is rocking back and forth rhythmically, to an insistent soundtrack that only he can hear. His hands are fists, his mouth is open, one foot is flopping against the other again and again and again. I am stalled in the doorway. I have never wanted to run away quite so much as I want to run away right now.

Dad talks to me. He says: 'Come in. Sit down.' He speaks gently, but it is not quite a request. 'Tell him you're here,' he says. 'Touch his arm. Show him you are here.'

Ben did not look how I expected him to. I had seen the long-term sick by this point, and I had noted in my callous way how the ailing body sometimes seems like something forgotten and perhaps badly stored, creased and dirty and worn away. My brother's body did not look like that. He was tall and slim and unblemished, a parody of wellness as he twitched and shuddered on the bed. I put a hand on his leg. I had not touched my brother in years, it seemed. We feel things in my family, great, untranslatable emotions, as are felt, I imagine, in every family. But we do not touch each other often. I only did it now because I did not want Ben to die.

Family love is the most complex, the most selfish. I needed Ben to live so that I could continue being myself.

And this: for all the years of adulthood I have often fretted tediously, indulgently, unconvincingly, about who I am. I have never wondered what I am, because I saw it there with Ben, lit up brightly in that accident of synapses. I saw what we all are, and I saw, at least I thought I saw, how easily we can be wiped away, even if it's only for a few minutes. The thing I now wonder about that day: where was Ben when we all gathered together in his bedroom? Was he still in there, looking out from some deep interior, unable to surface? Was he silently screaming as he shook back and forth? Or had he been taken somewhere else entirely? Had he been dropped down, muted, set to pause?

I think of Dad too. I wonder what he was thinking.

One of the most interesting things about having a child and watching them grow is seeing how things come online in stages. They can focus on you, then they can smile. They can hold their head up for themselves, then they can crawl. The brain of a newborn is not finished. For years it is growing, new pieces of it firing up as the months pass. Even now, this does not end. As I write this, my daughter is almost four years old, and yesterday she came in while I was reading, scarecrowed herself forcefully in front of the mirror and, looking down at her clothes, said: 'Does this *work*?'

Idiom, I noted to myself, and turned the page. What I should have noted was: imitation. I have done that a thousand times, asking Sarah before leaving the house whether it is okay to wear a checked shirt with checked trousers, if the checks, right, are of different sizes? I now understand that someone has been watching me, studying me, figuring out which stray bits of me to use as she constructs herself.

I also understand that sometimes things go offline in stages too. You lose one thing, and then a week later you lose another. Sometimes, like Ben, you get these things back. Sometimes, also like Ben, you do not.

It was a Christmas around the sagging middle act of my teens when my brother came home for the holidays to tell us that he had a brain tumour.

Except that's not quite right. That's how I now remember it, but then one crucial detail will contradict another, and over time I will realize that I do not know this story – my own family's story – as well as I think I do. Across the years, the version we all lived through has been compacted into the version we tell other people about – something that gets at the basic truth while ignoring the specifics. So let me think about this properly. Ben came home for the holidays, and he told us there was something wrong with him. And he told us not to worry about it.

It was 1994, I think, and I was busy failing a series of GCSEs. If I was sixteen, Ben would have been twenty-two. He seemed so old to me back then, but I now wince at the thought of having to do all that, face all that, when you're just twenty-two.

Tall and stylishly delicate, Ben was a stark icon of my childhood. He was a mystery, to me and to everyone else, which meant that he was endlessly interesting. He was a topic as much as a sibling. 'Your brother has this smile,' a friend of Ben confided in me once, possibly searching for more information, 'that suggests he knows things nobody else could ever know. It's an enigmatic smile. You could follow him around for twenty-four hours a day, every day of the week for ten years, and he'd still greet you with that smile.

'But I've worked him out,' Ben's friend continued. 'I know what his secret is.' I remember feeling my pulse flutter. My brother's friend shook his head. 'He's just a man who knows how to do an enigmatic smile.'

'I don't think that's quite it,' I said after a pause.

'Neither do I,' admitted my brother's friend.

I would never be like Ben, but at times I got tantalizingly close. We would say the same things at the same time, Ben and I. The world struck us both as being funny in the same way – or I learned to appreciate the mixture of mockery and sentimentality with which he approached life. I loved these moments of synchronicity, and I always longed for the next one, knowing, at the same time, that they cannot be fabricated or forced. They happen or they don't.

Ben had been away at college taking an access course for university when he started to have seizures, shaking him out of his seat in class and once launching him off his motorbike. These seizures were caused by a cyst, apparently. A pool of fluid inside the brain, pushing down against vital matter. An underground lake, dripping and unseen.

My family has spent twenty years trying to forget much of this period, but what we have actually achieved between us is an understanding that memory doesn't really work like that. It doesn't yield to pressure – and sometimes it stubbornly seems to dig in. I could go from any point in any conversation with any of my family to talk of Ben's illness, and nobody would register a segue: it remains, in rest, at the forefront of our minds. All I need to do is think of Ben, now middle-aged and living in Worcester and working in a library, and the whole thing comes back to me in a rush, memories stacked and loosed, like cards shuffled and then sprayed across the room. The seizures, the cyst, the night he told us all about it.

It was at Mum's house, which means we were chilly – another one of my mother's self-imposed struggles. She claims that she doesn't feel the cold, and if anyone turns a radiator on in her house, she mutters something about the war and rationing, even though she was born in 1949, and then she turns the radiator off again to improve us.

(And here's something parents can teach children: Mum taught me that I wanted to be a writer. One day in primary school, learning to read, we were all given flashcards with words – words like CAT and CAR and MOTHER. We had to go home and construct a few sentences. We were allowed to ask for help – and, man, I had help. Mum showed me that these basic, blameless units of language could be made to line up in interesting ways. I returned to school with something I still find pretty funny: MOTHER RAN OVER THE DOG.)

So we were sitting in the living room, watching our breath mist in the evening air, and Ben was idly handling one of the many detuned guitars he seems to leave behind him wherever he goes, a jangling wake. Even without the guitar, on the rare occasions that we get together, a family of our size inevitably looks like a band posing for a photograph, albeit an odd and not

enormously popular band. This particular moment would have
been a liner picture from a difficult second album.

I assume time has embellished much of this, because, honestly, it's almost a perfect memory: a dark Christmas snapshot,
glittering with detail. The cold, the house dithered into
shadow, lit only by glossy red candles and filled with holly my
mum had diligently stolen from nearby farms, and Ben telling
us about his head as he strummed softly and unmusically. The
cyst was in a good spot, apparently, between the brain and
the skull. *Easy to access* was the phrase he used, uttering the
words with the slightest hint of a laugh. He told us the cyst was
about the size of a fig. A pain, but nothing more. A solution
would be imminent.

How did we react? We scattered our own ways without
questions. Mum retreated into Radio 4. I went out to a movie.
And yet, wordlessly, something had been agreed upon. There
was an unspoken agreement between all of us: we were deciding not to give this information the time it needed. It was as if
we had received a coded message from an interesting source,
and had chosen not to decrypt it.

I assume everybody was as confused as I was, confused and
somehow affronted. I was baffled that these catastrophes really
happened to ordinary people, and with little sense of an appropriate thematic build-up. Our lives seemed too small-scale and
domestic for anything so shamelessly dramatic to explode
around us. It felt uncanny too. It was impossible to think back
on a decade or more of memories and now imagine the cyst
there with us, secretly pooling the whole time.

We stumbled away from that Christmas, and the planning
began. Treatment. Drainage? Lots to plan for. And then things
started to change. I remember us waiting. Waiting through a
clear perversion of pregnancy. The cyst was a fig. Then it
was an orange. Then it suddenly wasn't a cyst any more and

someone was explaining to us – always us, I have refused to accept any solitary memories – that tumours came in four grades, and grade four was the worst. This was a two.

It was an astrocytoma, so named because it grows from cells called astrocytes that live in the brain and spinal cord, and I gather it once struck someone that these cells look like stars. (Astrocytomas are a form of neuroglia, incidentally, cells which you could think of as being the caretakers of the nervous system, quietly keeping things ticking. I only mention this because the word *neuroglia* has a truly wonderful translation. It means 'nerve glue'.)

There was little time to think. Medical crises seem to borrow the rhythm of wartime, frantic action punctuating an endless period of waiting in which minds are left blank and useless, in which heads are ducked in readiness for the next shell that will fall. In spring, Ben had surgery in a pretty town just outside of Brighton that I have hated ever since. The surgery lasted for an afternoon and then long into the evening, and my imagination, strung out on endless comfort Dime bars, busily filled in the details for me, replacing the battered workaday blandness of hospital equipment with extravagant futuristic horrors. In the ICU I imagined Ben twisting, slowly, within a thick gel, stiff little bubbles frozen around him. In the operating theatre, *Mars Attacks* cannons, bulbous and heavily riveted, were trained on the back of my brother's skull. A slow, *Buck Rogers* execution.

Throughout all of this, though, I had a different vision of what was happening too, a competing schema that required no imaginative effort at all. The books in our house, the books Ben and I had grown up with, all of them were about islands. *Treasure Island*, *The Coral Island*, *Robinson Crusoe*, even *The Lord of the Flies*, which we both would have stumbled away from in English class around thirteen or fourteen, bludgeoned by that unflinching glimpse of Piggy's head, cracked open, with 'stuff' coming out of it. Islands were a place you got stuck sometimes, a place where you awaited rescue. Inevitably, unbidden, I thought of Ben on an island, long body stark against the sky, head bowed as he kicked over stones on the shoreline. Dad once told me that the Latin for island was *insula*. He was talking about *Don Quixote*, his favourite book, in which Sancho is promised the governance of an island for his loyalty and hard work. I suddenly grasped the origin of the word *insular*, and thought: That's perfect. An island is the perfect place for that special kind of loneliness, that inward journey.

Where was Mum? Rattling urgently between Kent and East Sussex in her Morris Traveller, fulfilling tiny but crucial missions that involved new books and clean clothes, all of it part of a wider campaign to remain busy and avoid thinking. It's how I would have handled things if I'd been in that position. Dad stayed put with Ben. And when Ben was in surgery, Dad looked after me, which meant sitting next to me in a car park in Sainsbury's while I cried. I can still remember the cool weight of his hand on my spine. I would think of it in the early days with Leon, when I would rub her back to ease her to sleep. To attain this kind of calm, Dad had become an expert. He had learned everything he could about cysts, and then he had to learn everything he could about tumours. It was a relief to me to have someone I could ask difficult questions – someone who knew me, and knew how to give me difficult answers.

My feeling back then was that Ben floated through all of this. Watching him each day in hospital in the lead-up to surgery, the reality of the situation seemed at times not to register with him. He just played cards, endless rounds of solitaire, and read thick books about Stalin.

Clearly, I completely missed the more complex emotional dimension. I missed Ben's anger, although I have since been told that he was so furious he wouldn't even talk to his doctors, leaving Dad to do the mediation. My brother wouldn't really talk to Dad either. In the few days before he went into hospital, Ben communicated with Dad via notes spelled out in the magnetic letters stuck to the door of the fridge at home. Basic notes, a warning that an emotion was spiking, perhaps, or a fragment of something lurid and brittle. One afternoon he left just two words: HELP ME. There wasn't room for much else. It was a small fridge.

I missed the fear too, and it's this that I really regret. I regret being unable to at least try to comfort my brother, and I also regret missing the opportunity to get to know him a little better. It is one thing to say things at the same time as another person. But it is something else to be able to understand why they are saying them. Ben was the kind of older brother who never really let you see the wheels going around. He was stylish and a bit of a rake and subject to a great deal of what media professors might refer to as the female gaze. In the strange, archaic grammar school that I attended in his wake, he was a legend, albeit for reasons that nobody could entirely pin down. I was always Donlan's brother there, although I would try to argue that I was also Donlan in my own right.

I didn't convince anybody about that one. Even the headmaster was in on it, a lofty public-school parody who walked the corridors wearing an academic gown and carrying a cup and saucer, and who had a harpsichord and a key to the city of St Petersburg in his office. He would squint and look faintly pained whenever my brother's name came up. 'Oh, Ben Donlan, yes,' he would say, as if being forced to recall a rare and distressingly poisonous type of frog that had once been found in his garden. 'He was very "cool", wasn't he?'

If I passed up the chance to comprehend this mysterious character a little more deeply in his suffering, I at least gained an understanding of the way that illness can change people in the most obvious ways. The day after his surgery, I went to see Ben in hospital, harbouring a real uncertainty as to what I would find. What does someone look like after brain surgery? Ben looked pretty relieved, actually: laughing, perhaps a little too loudly and a little too easily, and eating a grey hospital yogurt as we gathered around his bed in the neurological ward. He had plasters where the surgeon had drilled into his skull in order to fix a frame in place, however, and he had a horseshoe scar, clean and geometrical in its arc, cut into his scalp, which had been clipped down to stubble. That curving scar seemed inappropriately beautiful: a mugging by Euclid. You don't expect such elegance to accompany such violence. It did not even look like violence.

Most interestingly, a day after surgery Ben was still attached to something. I don't know what it was exactly, but a tube came out of the top of him, either carrying thick brown liquid away from the scar or feeding it in. It didn't seem right to ask which it was, and besides, I was done with finding out about the brain for the time being.

I have since read a little about brain surgery, and I'm glad that I was ignorant back then. I wonder how much Ben knew, going in.

Brain surgery: beyond the idioms, it's alarming to discover what a physical process it often is: reinforce this, remove that, stop all these things from rupturing. Yes, it's delicate, but largely because the brain is delicate. It's delicate in the way potholing is delicate: you're headed somewhere dangerous and cramped, and you don't want to do anything awful along the way. But still, potholing is not a dainty thing.

The tumour did not return in Ben's case, but he was changed by what had happened. He had fits due to scarring on the brain, and the drugs he needed to handle his fits created a kind of dampening effect, a very slight dulling of the wit, leading to a clumsiness in speech that I have recently come to recognize in myself too. I now know that Ben also lost the next five years, maybe more. He was convinced that he was going to die regardless of what he did.

This experience was never part of the past for Ben, but it became part of the past to me. And then, four or five years later, in my last year at university, a call in the middle of the night and it all started up again. Ben had begun to fit once more. He had lost the ability to speak. When asked, in hospital, to raise his right hand, his left leg shot out instead.

There was no regrowth of the tumour – Ben's neurosurgeon came out of retirement to confirm it on the new scans. This was just an incident, apparently. And then, four years later, another one, and much worse.

I was out of university this time and, stuck in an aimless job that wouldn't miss me, I went to stay with Ben and his wife while we tried to work out what kept going wrong – with the understanding that *we* would not be doing much of the working out. Again, Ben had lost the ability to speak. Again, his arms and legs did not respond correctly to instructions.

This time always strikes me as being the hardest time, even though, once again, the scans showed the tumour had not returned. When asked, Ben admitted that maybe he had been experimenting with not taking his medicine, but it was tricky to get a straight answer, and even trickier to understand what he said anyway.

Selfishly, it was the hardest time for me because I was ostensibly an adult now, and I should not be hidden from things any more, even if that's all I really wanted. That's why Dad took me in to see Ben fitting in his bedroom, creating a memory that I still do not entirely understand the meaning of.

Meaning is loose with things like this, anyway. By the time

of Ben's second relapse, I had read various books on the brain, perhaps in an unconscious effort to reclaim the brain from the frightening muddle of Ben's illness. It was thin protection against what was to follow, knowledge. Popular science meant I had great anecdotes and a blunt caricature of the mind, but here was the brain going wrong in front of me, contorting somebody I knew into somebody I didn't.

Again, selfishly – and it has always been hard for me not to be selfish around disease, even if it is someone else's – Ben's illness became a boundary for me: an upper limit to my own fear and even my own imagination when it came to considering the worst thing that could ever happen to a person. What could be more awful than a tumour beneath the skull, than the notion that death is alive inside you, and blooming? What could be worse than a limpet, attached to your brain and exerting a wet, subterranean pressure?

It was a boundary in another way too. The day after I saw Ben fitting on the bed in that new house of his, we all went back to the hospital together. Ben's daughter had just been born. He was the first of the Donlan children to have children of their own.

Ben was in and out of hospital a lot around the time his daughter was born, sometimes as a father, sometimes as a patient. As a father, his life was beyond me. I would not have understood what he was doing if I had taken years off to study it. As a patient, he spent a number of days in the medical assessment ward, a long, grumbling triage room where all kinds of patients flowed together, regardless of their situations.

I remember finding the doctors in this ward fascinating. The one in charge was short and puddingy and restless, racing from bed to bed with the names – or probably conditions – of each patient written on Post-it notes he had arranged on the waxy

cuffs of his old black work suit. He was forever moving them
around, those notes, updating them, crossing something out
with a blunted felt tip. Occasionally he would pluck a note off
his cuff and crumple it with a quiet kind of theatre: it meant
that someone had been moved upstairs. You could almost see
the space in his mind being freed for the next note, the next
patient. I sensed at the time he would not have crumpled a note
in a case where somebody had actually died. He presumably
had pockets to deal with that.

The doctor who really stood out, though, was Ben's
neurologist – the first neurologist I ever encountered. I remember thinking: You don't look like a neurologist – and then
wondering why I was so sure about that. In my mind, neurologists resembled the kind of German scientists who you'd see
designing new Audis in adverts. I knew what *glasses* a neurologist should wear: wire arms, no frames around the lenses. This
man looked like a landscape gardener, crumblingly handsome
in that English way and dressed the colours of autumn in a
shapeless woollen jumper and the sort of checked shirt Paddy
Ashdown wore to explain to the electorate that he was posh but
not frivolous.

This was the man who, behind the scenes, was organizing all
the scans and tests Ben was having: an MRI, which I pondered
with a kind of awe; and an 'LP', which ended up scrawled on
his notes one evening, scheduled for the next morning. 'Lipid
profile,' I reassured everyone, with the certainty of the very
stupid. 'Just a blood test. Nothing to worry about.' It was a
lumbar puncture, inevitably: not just a blood test, and very
much something to worry about.

Why this man has stayed with me, and why I think he would
have stayed with me even if my life didn't take some of the
turns it has subsequently taken, was that I got to see the way he
worked. And the way he worked was entirely unexpected.

He would hover by Ben, and just watch as Ben slid in and out of sleep.

It turned out that he watched Ben far more closely than the rest of us did. At one point, Dad was explaining to him that Ben had these fits, see, and the neurologist said rather mildly, 'Oh, look – he's having one now.' We all turned, and Ben *was* having one, rocking back and forth on his bed, mouth open. The neurologist nodded: he'd seen all he needed. The angle of Ben's head was important, he explained. I gather that it told him where the lesions probably were. He looked at Ben's charts, scribbled out the current medication and wrote in something else. The fits stopped after this, but a lot of our anxiety went away before we even started to understand that, somehow, he had just fixed everything.

Mine went away with, 'Oh, look – he's having one now.' To this man, Ben's fits were not a sign of the world collapsing inwards. They were useful. They aided him in some private, professional manner.

And he did all this just by looking. The neurologist is the person who sees. I would hear echoes of this idea the deeper I got into the world of neurology. But I saw it all there, right at the start, perfectly expressed in this contained, horticultural man with his lumpy jumper. The man who sees – and more than that, the man we have implicitly trusted to have seen everything already.

This, I realized after my first jolt of Lhermitte's in February, was who I needed. I needed a neurologist, a person who would be able to study me and look beneath my surfaces: beneath the skin and bone, but also beneath the hedging, the fudging, the inevitable bargaining. This impulse sent me to my GP, located down one of Brighton's more whimsical side streets, in the hinterland where last century's sunburnt crusties meet this century's whipcord dandies. It can be hard in a street like this to tell whether the gathering of a sinister throng means you're going to witness inept fist fights or a flash mob performing *Aida*. Quiet and drawn in close, I sat in the waiting room, a man slightly out of time among the Janets and the Barbaras, the occasional Arthur. Blood tests were scheduled and various bland possibilities were suggested, but for now I was diagnosed with a likely vitamin D deficiency, which didn't seem too bad, really. After the energy of Lhermitte's, I felt briefly short-changed.

I filled my prescription at the chemist's outside work: small turquoise pills, little rubbery gems filled with a clear liquid. 'Pure sunshine,' said the chemist, as he handed them over. 'Some days it feels like they're all I really dispense any more.'

Pure sunshine, but as winter edged towards spring a cloudiness was setting in again. My new-found calmness was spreading a little too far. At home, I was becoming vague, dawdly, prone to staring into space. 'Why did you draw sunbeams on your prescription stub?' asked Sarah one evening, hunting for change for the takeaway driver. Everything was starting to sound like a non sequitur.

'Sunbeams?' I asked, and Sarah showed me a small square of light green paper, with VITAMIN D printed at the top and a sun, drawn in orange highlighter pen, radiating heat beneath it. 'I think the guy at the chemist drew that,' I said.

'Weird,' said Sarah, while I continued to stare at the prescription, wondering if it had in fact been me who drew the sun.

I took the pills, and I did feel a little chirpier. And yet I knew. I knew that vitamin D was not the answer. The things that were going on inside me felt too big to be resolved by small, rubbery pills. Within a week I was back at the GP's anyway. The Lhermitte's had increased in force, and my GP announced it was time to see a neurologist.

I was referred in early March, and I soon had an appointment

booked for May. I had only two months of limbo in total: a
marvel of medical progress, given the history of neurological
illness, which extends wearily through entire lives, and min-
gles at times with the histories of witchcraft and demonic
possession and the things that get done to people who are suspected of falling foul of that sort of stuff. I had time to fill,
though, so I had a plan. Almost an anti-plan. I would not look
for myself online. I would not head to Google or WebMD. I
would not try to use my time, as I waited for my neurologist,
to become an amateur kind of neurologist myself. This was
cowardice, but cowardice delivered with a certain theoretical
rigour. I have always understood that when there's nowhere to
go, it's probably best to go nowhere.

And I did. When I think of those long spring weeks, it seems
that I spent almost the entire time on the 27, a bus that travels
between Westdene and Saltdean, two cheerily unimportant
suburbs on either side of Brighton and Hove. Nothing is quite
so prosaic as a trip by bus, and yet nothing has the same hyp-
notic capacity to gently transform either. I am a king when it
comes to falling asleep on the top deck, towards the rear, and I
am never quite the same person when I get off a bus that I was
when I got on.

This is all especially true of the 27, a route that, strictly
speaking, doesn't really go anywhere, describing a higgledy
loop into Brighton and then out again. There is a poetry to it,
regardless. Much of this journey takes you along the coast road
where, on the right kind of day, a churning sea meets throbbing
clouds, while the safety fencing bucks and wriggles along the
crumbling edge of the white cliffs for miles and miles. It's
almost a shock when the coast opens up like this. Brighton is a
cramped place full of limited horizons. Suddenly, out here, the
sky and the sea erupt around you. It's blinding.

I normally take the 27 from my home in Saltdean into work.

Now, though, I took it and stayed on past the regular stop – past any stops – as the bus obligingly arced me back and forth for dozens of empty-headed hours. I was not avoiding work, just as I was not avoiding my family: I diligently answered emails, and Leon was often with me, shaken to sleep by the engine. I was simply starting to realize that I was changing in ways I did not understand, and the bus seemed to provide a little breathing space while that happened. Riding the 27, as the wheels met the tarmac, my internal vibrations were cancelled – or rather universalized. Everyone else suddenly had them too.

It was time well spent, I think. Aimless and on a bus bound for nowhere, I found myself thinking about exploration, about movement into uncertain territories, about guides, and how clear it was that I needed one. I thought about the neurologist, who I hoped would soon make sense of my symptoms (and possibly even dismiss them: another alarmist, another time-waster).

On the day before I saw my neurologist, I told Sarah that the only way through any of this was to get right to the point. I would learn from Ben, and I would not be angry. I would be upfront about my fears, and I would say, in effect, just two words: *Help me.*

The next day I returned to the neurological ward just outside Brighton that I had last visited when I was sixteen and my brother was having brain surgery. The place had barely changed, a bright sprawl of corridors, separated from the main hospital and accessed via two flights of stairs, down, down, down. Inside, it was cool and airy despite the sense, after all that descending, of being deep underground. And it was so muddling in its branching hallways and dead ends that its navigational challenges seemed born of a desire to mirror the shifting, confusing landscape of the neurological patients themselves.

Like so much of the modern NHS, there was a pluckiness to

this building. An immediate jolt of Blitz spirit you felt as soon as you entered it. The whole place was like a 1940s code-breaking installation churning in the basement of the hospital. Why not? Both neurologists and cryptanalysts are dealing with an enemy that is hard to anticipate. Both are working with imperfect information. And at the centre of it all?

His name is not Quill, but that will have to do. Quill is as close as I can get you to him without sacrificing either his deli-cate, scrupulous nature or his privacy. Quill will do.

And Quill is a riddle, or at least he sounds like one whenever I try to describe him. He seems like an extremely tall person to me, even though he is actually around my height, so entirely average. I remember him as unduly thin, and he is not – not particularly thin, anyway, just *average*, like me. Equally, I get the sense he is witty, but he has hardly had a reason to try to make me laugh. Maybe I am simply responding to his evident quickness, to a mind that darts.

Like many specialists, he seems to have come from a differ-ent era: a young Victorian. Most confusing of all, he is one of the most important people in my life, and yet I have met him on only a handful of occasions, and spent less than an after-noon, all told, in his company.

Much of this is transference, I am sure, but I felt it almost immediately: a rush of grateful attachment. As I think back on my first meeting with Dr Quill, deep in the scramble of the neurology wards, I can't help but project things into the mem-ory. I can't seem to leave the thought of Quill alone.

Quill was not initially that interested in what I had to say. I imagined we'd go straight to the question of a history, but the history came second. Quill was polite as he showed me in and found my file. He smiled at my nervous chatter, but he was focused largely on what I looked like and how I moved, and in the rhythm of speech rather than the content.

Quill's eyes are large, and they move around very quickly. The day I met him, he looked canny, capable and watchful – and gently, appealingly, awkward too. He seemed one of those men who forever struggle to hide the schoolboy they once were, wearing his shirt and tie like a uniform and in a manner that somehow made it clear that he would probably dress this way regardless of whether he was coming into the hospital or not. Yes, I liked Quill immediately, even as he then forced me through the gamut of twitchy dexterity challenges which I now understand are the diagnostic front line of neurology – the quickest way to get inside somebody else's head without drilling.

The most common observation made about neurological examinations is that they are a lot like roadside sobriety tests. In fact, they basically are roadside sobriety tests: walk toe-to-heel in a straight line, touch your nose with each finger in sequence, lean in and stare while a torch beam plays across your pupils. Having a neurological examination that day, I felt that I had been pulled over, in some manner of speaking. Everyone else got to race by on their business, but I must wait on the margins and fret.

What these tests are really telling you, though, is that the brain is hiding, and its secrets are not easy to get at. When I heard that I was about to have a neurology exam, I expected machines and scan lines, wires and electrodes and those sticky pads. I expected a direct communion with science, which for me meant technology. My brain would speak and the machines would listen and understand. In truth, it is all far more personal than that at first. The machines will come, but for now the doctor must watch and listen, must get at the brain through the brain's compromised vessel.

Finger-tapping, gaze-tracking, measurements of gait: I was subjected to a fierce and benign scrutiny that day. Doctors, almost alone among professionals, are allowed to really stare at other people, and the best of them indulge this allowance as much as they can. I failed many of the tests I was faced with in an amusing fashion, but I probably would have failed a lot of them even if I were entirely healthy. Quill managed to separate my innate lack of physical ability from genuine neurological clues.

Then, once we had sat down again, he finally leaned towards me and asked me how I was feeling right now. Doctors are allowed to do that too.

I launched into my tumour fears – fears that were announcing themselves to me even as I spoke them aloud. When I mentioned Ben's case, Quill made a note of it in tiny handwriting and asked what had happened. I explained that the tumour had been removed, and I could tell that, for a second, Quill was thinking about crossing Ben out entirely. Sensing the problematic symbolism of that, perhaps, he instead wrote something equally tiny next to his original note and drew a wonky line around it, walling it off from the rest of my history – present but now deemed irrelevant.

After that, I told Quill what I'd been telling Sarah for the last few months since January: that I just felt wrong and I didn't know what was happening to me. The world of touch had changed, and ever since that day in February when I met Sarah in the coffee shop, I now buzzed when I moved my head forward. I caught at this point a millisecond flash of recognition, a cataloguing impulse which was quickly and elegantly disguised, and then Quill asked me to continue. I told him that every day I had the sensation that things were spreading outwards, that fresh defences were falling and new territory was being lost. 'You feel like a battleground?' Quill asked me, and I laughed. I told him: I feel like a building that is slowly being burgled. Vital doors are breached, valuables are disappearing haphazardly, alarms going off that nobody else hears. If only I could keep track of what is being stolen.

'Go back,' he then said to me. He may have touched my arm to signal that this was important. 'What has the last year or so been like? Even before your hands started tingling. Anything strange?'

I went back. I tried to, anyway. I skimmed over my recent life, and didn't really see anything worth mentioning. I did not suspect that my door-handle problem might be connected – or that it was potentially even a problem rather than an amusing curio. I missed a strange morning, over a year ago, when I woke up in our old house and everything just ached. Sarah only remembered this long after the fact, when she was looking through her old search history and came across a flurry of inquiries into Hodgkin's lymphoma. Life is full of symptoms we ignore, or investigate briefly, only to set aside. Mine was, anyway.

Rather than presenting these details, which might have been useful, I came up with others that I assumed might be relevant, perhaps attempting to tilt things in the favour of a milder diagnosis. I mentioned Leon, who we carried around a lot at that age. I mentioned moving, with all those boxes that needed to go into the loft. Plenty of opportunities to damage a neck.

Quill nodded, politely, but I don't recall him noting any of these last musings down. Instead, before he booked me in for an MRI and scheduled another appointment to go over the results of that, he shuffled his papers and knotted his hands together. Long fingers, pale skin. A careful, slightly Holmesian meshing that seemed to verge on parody. Or perhaps experience had simply taught him that patients tended to need this sort of the-atre in a doctor.

'From a diagnostic point of view, I can't see anything wrong with you,' he said at last. 'All we have to go on is the things you say you're feeling, and that's good – that's good.' We smiled. But he wasn't finished.

'From what you're telling me, I think you have some kind of lesion on your cervical spine.' My eye started to twitch. This definitely sounded less good. Like most people, I am able to live with the knowledge that I have something as crucial and delicate as a spine only by ignoring the fact as much as possible. And now I had a cervix too.

And yet, at the same time as I was starting to worry again, I also realized that Quill was much more of a magician than I had expected him to be. My spine? All that from watching me pat my own head and walk across the room?

'There are three main reasons why it could be there,' he continued. 'You could have injured your neck somehow – it's true you have no symptoms above the neck?' I ticked off my catalogue of buzzes and aches: feet, legs, arms, fingers. He was right: nothing above the neck. 'So injury is definitely a possible cause. Then it's possible that you have inflammation in your spine as a one-off. Some people just get an inflammation and then it goes away.

'With some people, though, it turns out to be more serious than that.'

Looking back, it is all so obvious to me. He knew. He knew *instantly*.

I am going to be completely honest about this. Since I first heard about MRIs, I knew I was going to have one sooner or later. I knew that machine was for me.

Ben was obviously at the heart of this certainty. A desire to follow my older brother's path, regardless of the bucks and turns. This sounds ridiculous, but I have a clear memory of Ben in hospital, on one of his later relapses, being readied for an MRI as he sat on his bed. The doctor is filling out a form. Dental work? Piercings? Neither, says Ben. The doctor asks: 'Have you ever been in a magnetic field before?' And Ben answers, worldly, flirtatious even, 'Oh, yes.' *Ohhhh, yes.* I took note of that moment. The sheer weight of experience being expressed was intoxicating.

I was fascinated by these machines, looking like the time-tunnel apparatus in movies like *Twelve Monkeys* – or rather it's the time-travel apparatus in movies that looks like them. When I pictured Ben, lost in the process of his diagnosis, I almost always saw him in the half-light of an MRI interior, lying flat, hands held together gently on his stomach, staring at the ceiling that curves inches above his head. It always felt particularly lonely: this scenario seemed to speak most clearly to the way that, when we are ill, we are especially isolated from the rest of the world.

'What does it sound like?' I asked him once.

'It sounds amazing,' he said. 'It sounds like music in there.' Ben always liked odd music.

I do not expect this to be universal – in fact, it sounds completely insane – but I have often tangled MRIs up with love too. With love revealed for what it might truly be: lights firing in the darkness of the brain. And this association is Sarah's fault, I will argue. On an early date, desperate to appear unusual, I heard myself telling her of a magazine piece I had read about Parkinson's disease and algae. The algae was photosensitive and bioluminescent: it could be made to light up, and to react to light from elsewhere. The idea is that doctors would place little dopamine machines in the warm dark spaces of the Parkinson's brain, and they would use the light to trigger the machines to unleash their chemicals when required. No need for electricity, no challenge to the brain's delicate wiring. Sarah actually licked her lips at that, and I remember it: she was physically thrilled at the thought of someone whose interests were as medical as her own. And over time the memory twisted together with love and a notion of how thoughts in a brain were ripples of light in an MRI, blood flow suggesting syn-apses firing. Unseen in the darkness of the skull but perhaps answered, nearby, in the darkness of another skull.

And so my own MRI came around in June, outsourced by the NHS to an improbably fancy private hospital in the sticks: a commuter hotel with kidney bowls under the beds. Sarah and I lent Leon to her grandparents for the morning and took the bus together. The bus was delayed, and I was grateful for the rising panic that I would miss my appointment, because it stood in front of a greater panic – that I was about to climb inside a tube for the best part of an hour while a magnet more powerful than I could imagine focused its attentions on me to the extent that the protons in my body would all line up the same way.

Nasty set-up. You meet the radiologist, who will sit behind glass, seeing the scans as they appear in real time. You will not get to see these scans. This radiologist will be eager to tell you that they cannot read the scans themselves, which only makes you more certain that they *can* read the scans and they're just lying about it. On the way out, you will study the radiologist for any clues, any tells, to what they might have seen. What-ever expression they assume as you walk past will contain dark certainties.

But before that, the machine itself. There is something reli-gious about an MRI scanner. It has an otherworldly charisma, sitting vast and curvy in its own room. Voices dip. Everybody seems to tense up in proximity. You almost want to leave a trib-ute of some kind. Looking back on this – I have had several MRIs by this point, and when they ask me if I have ever been in a magnetic field before, I can now answer, *Ohhhh, yes*, for myself – I am always somewhat surprised that they are not surrounded by an annulus of eagle feathers and pine cones, rev-erently placed.

I am laid out on a gurney. Headphones are wedged over

my ears and a cage is clamped to my head. I feel that rush of panic I always get from enforced stillness. Then voices. Suddenly, there are two people standing over me, and I can see neither of them.

'Bertie is here,' one of the voices says. 'He wants to put in the needle.'

'Fine by me,' I say chirpily, while internally I am thinking: The *needle*?

'He hasn't done it before. It's training.'

'Okay!' I say, with exactly the same chirpiness, so that I sound insane.

There is fussing. A jab in my arm. Something cold starts to trickle down my elbow.

'Bertie only gets one go,' says the voice. 'I'll take over, Bertie.'

The needle is for contrast: they are dipping my brain in ink so that the MRI scanner will be able to see the damaged bits. And then I am rolled into the machine. Grey plastic curves overhead. It makes me think of the rounded plastic of aeroplane luggage lockers, except this is what they'd be like if you'd decided to enjoy long-haul travel from the inside of one. Aeroplanes feel right, in fact: that same sense of a suspended life I feel at take-off, that same sense of being apart from the rest of the world, of wondering how I got here, and wondering if I will be allowed to return.

The machine fires up. The sound is industrial, intensely loud. There is a sound of thudding, slamming, high-pitched whining, and a sort of stickiness, as of large things coming together and coming apart with wet reluctance. Music? More than anything else, MRI scanners sound like a factory involved in the large-scale production of syrup – a factory that has been constructed, for reasons best left unexplored, somewhere behind the bridge of your nose.

'Two-minute picture, hold still,' comes the voice in my ears. I love the use of the word *picture*, as if I am sitting for a daguerreotype. Ridiculously, I give a thumbs-up at this, and hit my hand against the roof of the tunnel I'm lying in. So far in! So narrow. Fighting back another moment of panic, and then we're away. The weird truth is that, on a purely sensory level, having an MRI is quite comforting – if you're an adult. The brain can't help but find rhythms within the alien sounds. For children, they pump in nursery rhymes – but who would want to think of a child in an MRI scanner?

I am aware, during all this, that I am becoming a map now. My head and spine are being cross-sectioned, so I am turning into those lagoons, ox-bows and bleached chalk tracks you see on the finished scans of strangers. Cross-sections of the head – medical cross-sections – always look the same to me: they always look like ridiculous flights of fancy, drawn by someone who has forgotten what a human head truly looks like. The brain is a hasty doodle. The eyeballs, suspended yolk-like for poaching, seem like an actual joke.

They call MRI scanners the Doughnut of Truth in this hospital, apparently, and it's a brilliant name. It helps explain to me the complex and highly charged feelings I have about them, the mix of grateful terror they manage to create. MRIs are a break from the business of having symptoms and then trying to describe them, trying to turn them into words. You cannot tilt the outcome of an MRI with words at all. You cannot argue with them – they are proof, a verdict.

All of this is suddenly clear to me as I finally roll out of the grey plastic tunnel after forty-five minutes. I blink, run a tongue around a mouth of dry, plasticky gums and someone else's teeth. I feel like I have been travelling, like I have landed and now must navigate a new set of customs and rituals. I feel, as well, like I have emerged from the machine but not from its shadow. I will feel it, looming, in the background for the next few weeks.

On the way out, I study the radiologist, who looks away. He seems to me to be smirking out of sheer animal awkwardness. Bertie is nowhere to be seen. Maybe this is Bertie.

A month later, in early July, a second MRI: more grey plastic, more alien sounds, more of Bertie and his cold contrast sliding up my arm. This time, it was part of a whole day of tests. An MRI in the morning and a lumbar puncture in the afternoon.

I had not worried sufficiently about the lumbar puncture: that was the problem, I realized, as I was led to a small room with a bed in it and a doctor preparing a range of needles.

In addition to not really worrying about the lumbar puncture, I had made two crucial mistakes in my preparation for it. I had done some research, and I had also done the wrong kind of research. Rather than reading up on lumbar punctures from a patient's point of view, which would have revealed that Dr Quill was interested to see what foreign bodies might be floating around uninvited in the fluid that surrounded my brain and spinal cord, I read up on the procedure from a practitioner's point of view, in which the patient is a raw material: fleshy, giving, but not giving too much. I read up, in essence, on how to deliver a lumbar puncture to myself.

Push the needle in until you feel the first resistance, I had read. Then push through that to a second resistance. First resistance! Second resistance! I was inside and outside at once: I was seeing the needle puncturing walls of clear flex and travelling through grainy human jelly, but I was also imagining the doctor, working by sensation alone, eyes closed for extra acuity. As if cracking a safe, as if reaching into a hole in a wall to grab for something nestled among sparking wires.

It seemed an improbably high-stakes affair, a needle in the

back. A needle going through territory that also held the delicate filaments of my spine, filaments I now instinctively understood were made of individual hairs of spun glass, sharp and fine and brittle. Fibre optics. The doctor tried to keep me talking as my panic rose. I lay down on the bed, turned away from her as directed, and held Sarah's hand, as Leon sometimes does when she is eager for sleep and knows she cannot get there alone. Again: things were happening that I could not see. A tap was being installed in my back, the needle working its way in between vertebrae.

'Video games? What's it like working on video games?' the doctor asked. Even now, even here, I could anticipate the next question. It was going to be: 'So you actually get paid to play games for a living?'

'I'm sorry,' I explained. 'I can't really think about that right now.'

Rude, and I'm sure I apologized at least once more in the moments that followed. And I felt that needle. I felt it huge, scaled up by my imagination so it was like a javelin going through me. I gripped Sarah's hand more tightly and dug in my fingernails. I felt a rush of nausea. 'You're turning a bit green,' Sarah said, and placed a hand on my forehead. 'It's just panic making you want to be sick.'

For whole minutes I felt sick, thought of wrenching myself away from the bed, pictured broken glass in my spine.

What rescued me from this moment was something very strange: pain. At one point, the doctor must have brushed the needle against a nerve, because the entire right side of my right leg suddenly ignited: the blinding white heat of a magnesium burn, making a nerve that ran from my groin to my toes announce itself in an instant with the tautness and bite of a piece of cheese wire. The whole thing just went up in one go. I contracted, but I also thought: That was interesting. Pain in my leg – real, tangible pain, suggestive of awful physical things which I know have not happened – caused by a needle in the back. Welcome to neurology! Welcome to neurology.

'Almost done,' said the doctor, a minute or so later. She held up a small vial of liquid. 'Nice and clear, good job.'

Stupidly, I felt proud.

Tests and the days in shadow between them. So much of my life seemed to bleed away as I moved between one MRI and the next. I ceased to do much in the way of meaningful work whenever I turned up at the office. Thankfully, I knew from the odd glance from my editor that they were aware something was up, but would wait for me to tell them about it. Most of my time at work was not spent writing about games, or even playing games. It was spent in the echoing hallway, out back and away from everyone, where private phone calls are made. I remember these moments very well, and even the memories of them conjure an old anxiety. On hold to a neurologist's secretary, the whole thing feeling somehow shady, filling me in some dull and persistent way with guilt. This distant world of specialists and their secretaries had suddenly drawn close. I might catch my reflection in a hallway window as I listened to hold music: this is my world now, or I am in their world now.

Luckily I was also in Sarah's world, and in Leon's world. We got away for a weekend to a cottage in Dorset that Sarah's parents were renting. Swanage, which had seemed like the most tedious place on earth when I had been there with my mum in my early teens. Now, though, it seemed beautiful: a perfect seaside town, somehow hidden from the rest of the world, accessible only via a rickety ferry and a wonderfully lonely drive down a desolate sand-blown road.

We stood on the flat roof of the place we were staying one night and looked across the bay. With Leon held in one arm and another around Sarah, I felt protected from everything, from whatever was going on inside, from the medical world that I knew was actually trying to help me.

'It's so weird being back around doctors,' I said to Sarah. 'I remember leaving the hospital when Leon was born and looking at the hallways, at the old furniture and the machinery, and thinking: This is great that this is all here, but I'll be glad to see the back of it for a while.'

'When was your last experience of it before that?' Sarah asked.

I had to think about it. 'God, it was years ago. I'd just turned thirty.' I had been on the Bone Marrow Registry for a decade before that, and then I'd had a call one afternoon that there had been a match. I'd gone into hospital for a day and given someone a bag of my stem cells. It had been the best thing I had ever been involved with — although Sarah and Leon had since replaced it.

'You've done all right,' said Sarah, as Leon stirred and I checked, now instinctively, on the state of her nappy. 'To get Leon in the bag, to get that in the bag, before anything went wrong.'

'Is it going wrong now?' I asked.

Sarah smiled and said nothing, and we went in for dinner.

Days later, I was back in Brighton, and back with Dr Quill. Some tests were in; others were still waiting to be interpreted. We were gathered in the same room as before, but it was afternoon, golden imprints of sunlight edging along the walls in slow arcs.

Quill waited until I was seated, and then leaned forward on his chair, hands together in his lap. 'You have an inflammation of the spine,' he said, possibly aware that I would have no idea what this meant. 'And we're trying to work out why. Some people have inflammation in the spine and it just goes away, like I said.'

'And then there are the other people?' I asked.

'Some people have it because they have multiple sclerosis.'

Something inside me seemed to fall away as he said this. A structural crumbling, rather than a smash: silent clouds of dust rushing outwards. A million miles passing in one soft second.

'Multiple sclerosis,' I replied. I sensed a question was expected of me, but I could not seem to form one. 'Multiple sclerosis.'

'Yes.' Quill nodded. He peered at me, watchful as ever, searching for some sign of understanding. 'Do you know what that is?'

'No,' I laughed eventually. 'I have absolutely no idea.'

'Multiple sclerosis,' Sarah says that night as we sit in bed, Leon snoring next to me, a clammy hand on my shoulder. It is a warm July evening, so the windows are open and the smell of cut grass drifts in from the green. 'Mul-tiple scleroooosis.' She is trying the words out, getting a sense of them in the lips, in the mouth.

'That was your first guess,' I say. 'Two minutes in. I wake up with funny hands and you diagnosed me while half asleep.'

She gives me a look that says: Now is not the time to bring this up.

And she works her way closer to me. 'We will deal with this,' she says. 'We will get through it.' She squeezes my hand. 'It may be nothing, and if it's not nothing,' she sighs, 'well, if it's not nothing, it's a big thing, isn't it? And we can always deal with the big things.'

Minutes later, as she starts to drift off, I ask: 'Will this kill me?'

'Probably not,' says Sarah. An offhand answer, perhaps, but by this point I have been firing idiotic questions her way for the best part of an evening. 'It probably won't kill you *directly*,' she clarifies. 'It may just lead to something that eventually does kill you.' Her eyes rest on me here. A tilt of the head. An appraising gaze that I cannot meet for too long. 'You'll probably die of pneumonia.'

This cheers me up. I know nothing about pneumonia, and I find that, as a result, I have little fear of it.

Soon Sarah is asleep. I sit in the dark and think of Ben. He was on that island for years. But the tumour was resected. The relapses died away. He got back to the mainland, more or less. He escaped.

Could I? I pull out my computer and type the words into Google for the first time. *Multiple sclerosis*. A sense of how the words feel in the fingers, how they feel beneath the hands. A minute later, I shut the laptop and put it on the floor. In the meantime I have watched the beginning of a YouTube video in which a woman with MS tries to explain what MS is like.

She tries. Her voice is a gargling mess, a choking, backed-up sink of a thing. Her eyes shine, bright and wet. They stare *out* at me somehow, as if from a very deep setting in her head. A tunnel lies between the both of us, and she is daring me to look away.

Phineas Gage, the Most Famous Neurological Patient in History

On a warm afternoon over a century and a half ago, Phineas Gage and his doctor took a stroll together along the banks of the Black River, just outside the small town of Cavendish, in Vermont. Gage gathered pebbles as they walked, selecting any that were bright enough or smooth enough to take his fancy. Soon he had collected a jiggling dozen or so: an enduringly pleasant thing to have, a handful of pebbles.

Before the two men parted ways, something odd happened. Gage's doctor offered to buy the collected pebbles for one thousand dollars. Gage refused. And he was furious: furious with his doctor at the thought of being cheated like this. Phineas Gage was a neurology patient, arguably the most famous who has ever lived. The matter of how much Gage's pebbles were worth was the first indicator that he would never be cured, that he would for ever be changed. It was the first indicator that his old self was out of his grasp for good.

Not that he would have understood this. Gage was a construction foreman who had had the misfortune to blast a metre-long iron pole through his own head, destroying much of his brain's left frontal lobe. The accident occurred in 1848, a year in which gleaming ribbons of train track were arcing across America, in constant need of people to clear the rocks from their paths to keep them moving. Gage was the boss of a demolition

crew working in Vermont, and one day he was uncharac-
teristically careless while setting a dynamite charge. His
tamping iron – the metre-long pole at the centre of this
story, which weighed about six kilograms – may have
struck the side of the boulder that he was rigging, creating a spark that prematurely set off the explosive. It is
impossible to focus too closely on thoughts of what happened next, but after the short journey through Gage's
skull, entering via the roof of his mouth and leaving
through the very top of his head, the pole landed some
nine metres away. Gage was knocked flat on his back.

   And then he sat up.

   Gage survived, but was transformed. A formerly kind
and decent man, after a lengthy period of recovery he
apparently became ornery, sly and somewhat dangerous
to be around. The frontal lobe is associated with
reward, attention, planning and motivation: the complex
business of managing self-interest during social interactions, among other things. Damage to this area left
Gage disinhibited – a compact and precise word carrying
lavish, cartwheeling implications. It also helped propel
him into the centre of arguments already raging in the
study of the brain and its relationship with the mind:
arguments between one group of people who believed
the brain was a single unit, all of it working as one piece
to create thought, and another group who believed that
the brain was divided into modules, localized areas with
bespoke purposes.

   Confusingly, both sides of this debate felt Gage was
clinching the case for them. The whole-brainers saw
Gage's survival as proof that the brain could compensate
for the loss of any individual part. The localizers, however, saw his survival as proof that the brain could handle

the loss of certain modules, depending on their functions. By and large, the localizers were correct, even if they were wrong about the places they chose to locate specific modules. The whole-brainers were correct about the brain's inherent interconnectedness, however, and they also may have foreseen the brain's plasticity – the manner in which one part of the brain can, given time, change its function to compensate for a deficit elsewhere.

More importantly to a newly minted neurology patient like me, the message of Gage's life is that neurological events change people – and that some change must be expected. Gage's conversion from dependable professional to swearing, cheating reprobate suggested that the brain might control aspects of character and behaviour to the extent that damage to a certain region could fundamentally alter a person's humanity. It strongly suggested that what was human in a person in the first place was probably stored inside their skull.

Equally, Gage's subsequent employment as a stage-coach driver in Chile, a job that seemed to have rehabilitated him, or at least curbed his most problematic new traits, hinted at how creating structure in the lives of the gravely brain-damaged might help them. Gage's gruesome accident touched upon the central realities of modern neuroscience, in other words, and also revealed the potential for treatment. It tells us that the brain is powerful and fragile, and that it is also highly adaptable.

What a life. Photographs of Gage depict an almost comically handsome character with high cheekbones and a strong jaw. Put him in a cape and he would be Superman, were it not for the permanently closed left eye, and the somewhat brittle bearing that is suggested as he clutches the tamping iron in his huge hands. It is sad, I think, to see him brandishing the object that caused him so much pain – his fate, and his fortunes, for ever linked to the worst thing that happened to him.

Gage died in 1860, aged just thirty-six. Still, in his fumbling, wretched way, he helped change the world. Over the years, historians and neurologists have argued about the specifics of his accident and recovery as well as the wider lessons to be learned from his case, and yet, perhaps due to his diminishing historical context, Phineas Gage remains the patron saint of neurological patients.

And I realize now that, standing on the border of the neurological world, I was looking for something very specific from Gage when I first started reading about him. I was looking for someone like me: someone who had a problematic brain. But I was also looking for someone far worse off than me, a person whose experiences I would never match, but who might still give me context.

I was looking for someone who had endured something I knew I wouldn't have been able to, and who was still sufficiently engaged with life afterwards that they wanted to seek out the prettiest pebbles they could find, and hold on to them.

4. The Frankenstein Dance

Leon learned to eat. Broccoli. Apples. The first ground to a gritty paste in her gappy Popeye mouth, eyes registering the pepperiness that the rest of us no longer noticed. The second huge and glossy in her soft hands, juice blending with saliva as she scored the powdery white flesh with emerging teeth, laughing at the tartness, the vividness of first fruit.

And she learned to speak. *Momma. Dadda. Apple.* The bright elements of her expanding world were coming into focus.

For both these tricks *learning* is the wrong word. It does not capture the wild cognitive leaps involved. In truth, Leon taught herself. No, in truth, one day she realized that she already knew how to do these things and so she simply began to do them.

Learning to eat, learning to make noises. This is basic stuff, I know, but still: the darting of her eyes, the eagerness of her mouth to register surprise in the form of a smile lifted all of this somewhat. Leon was changing, transforming from a newborn into something a little more advanced and substantial. A different person was emerging, outlined by her new abilities, prosaic as they would seem to everyone but Sarah and me.

Transformation was in the air. In the first week of July, fresh from the MRI tube, I went with my friend Simon to see a new exhibition on digital art at the Barbican in London. Simon had interviewed one of the artists involved the day before and wanted to see the finished thing; I was largely propelled by an eagerness to get away from the office, where I was having all of my NHS mail sent, each fresh envelope an indicator that there was nothing wrong with certain parts of my brain at least, judging by the jolts of fright they were still capable of delivering.

On the train up, Simon told me about this artist of his and I tried to listen: videos for Kanye and Arcade Fire, work in galleries in LA and New York. And this time he'd appropriated an awkward and flighty motion-sensing camera from a video game console, a device that could track people's movements and do interesting things with the data. Installation art.

'I think you'll like it,' Simon said, as we entered the gorgeous ashtray gloom of the Barbican itself. I asked him to sign me in at the reception desk, after seeing how narrow the lines ruled in the press book's pages were. He raised an eyebrow but did as I asked. 'Something's up with my hands,' I muttered. Something was. They fizzed and sputtered as we walked into the darkness of the exhibition, dying sparklers attached to each of my wrists.

This artist of Simon's had done something extraordinary. After a few rooms of every video game cliché in the world – stacks of dead consoles yellowing on metal shelving, Mario running and jumping on cutting-edge HD monitors that robbed him of the classic Valium haze he assumed on the old home telly – we turned a corner and found ourselves in a long dark chamber with a wall of pure white light at the far end of it. The chamber was tall, high-ceilinged and cold, a churchy echo gathering in the quiet air above us.

One by one, the people in front of us stood before the wall of light, where there was a form of shadow theatre in play, picking out each person as a fidgety silhouette, and then tracking them as they moved between three panels of blinding white emptiness.

In the first panel, people were still coming to terms with their projected silhouette. They would reach out their arms

and splay their fingers. The shadow they cast was eager to fragment, however: black shards turning into birds that scattered
into the sky and left nothing behind.

When they moved to the second panel, the shadow returned.
But so did the birds, this time wheeling down out of the rafters
to pull this new shadow to pieces, tearing and ripping and disappearing with jagged wet chunks of flesh.

If they could handle the final panel they would discover
that the shadow was back again, but the birds were nowhere to
be seen. Not at first, anyway. Now, when people spread their
arms, they grew wings, their sudden appearance accompanied
by a great corrugated flapping sound. Silhouette wings with
depth, with articulation, with individual feathers fanning out
sharply from the wrists to the armpits. It was shocking, the
best kind of shock: first sombre and then delightful. Despite
the almost-religious ambience of the high room and the pools
of darkness, people invariably laughed when they saw their
own wings, even if they absolutely knew what was coming.

'It's beautiful,' I said to Simon afterwards, both of us sitting
in a coffee shop deep beneath the shadow of the looming Barbican. 'I don't get how he got it all so right,' I said. 'That sense of
being torn apart by something beautiful' – Simon started to
smile as I continued, hunting for the words – 'by something so
filled with life. And so *necessary*.'

Simon, elegant and inscrutable, raised an eyebrow again, perhaps connecting my extreme emotional response – something
that was clearly a confused, private reading of simple public
art – to my inability to sign the register an hour before.

I realized too late that I wasn't talking about the installation
any more. So I told Simon about the tests I was having, about
the tingling in my hands and feet, about the slow dawning
of the fact that I was having trouble walking long distances
now, that my world was starting to shrink. And I told him

about my last meeting with Quill, and those words of his: *multiple sclerosis*.

Simon did that thing I have since discovered that people do. His face managed to move without moving, a kind of internal settling to accommodate the news. Then Simon shook his head. A long moment passed. 'Weirdly, of all the diseases you could get, I would have picked you for this,' he said at last. He then immediately considered what he had just said. 'Well, I wouldn't *pick* you for this, but I mean, it fits.'

I laughed. 'Really?'

'You've always loved all that neurology stuff,' he said. 'There was that thing you told me about memory a while back.'

That thing I told him. Of course he loved that. I had half-read somewhere that memory isn't just open to distortion, but that it positively runs towards it. It craves embellishment and fabrication. Each time you remember something, you pull down the volume you're after, you read it, and then you destroy that volume and rewrite it. That is memory. Remembering something is an act of destruction, covered up by an almost-instantaneous act of creation. But this is a compromised creation: it is a forgery, a copy of something that is almost certainly a copy of something already. The life behind us shifts around just as much as the life ahead of us.

And I do like that fact, as it happens. I do like to read about what thinking is, ponder what thoughts themselves might be made of. But Simon was wrong on a deeper level: I like thoughts, but I do not love brains. After all, I have never really liked the fact that I have a brain.

And suddenly I realized I was still with Simon beneath the Barbican. I had not spoken in a while. I changed the subject, asking him about his daughter, who was about to switch schools, moving from primary to secondary, from a school a few streets away to a school at the end of a train ride. Simon was worried: her friends were all going elsewhere.

'This is an opportunity in disguise,' I argued, complacent in the knowledge that my own daughter would not have to go to school for years. 'Everything changes at eleven. Here's a chance for her to reinvent herself.'

Simon looked unconvinced. 'You know,' I continued, 'a chance to recast something difficult as something beneficial, to be the new person she wants to be.'

I recognized, too late, that I was talking about myself again. But I also recognized that there was something to this: something to the idea that my disease – whatever it might be – could be an opportunity as well as a catastrophe. A chance to explore, to step away from an old identity and towards another one, even if I had not entirely chosen the next one myself.

Quill had given me hope, if I wanted it. *No symptoms above the neck?* he had asked. This meant it could all be down to an injury, or a single lesion on the spinal cord. I sensed at the time, though, that he did not think these things were very likely. I also sensed that I did not think them very likely either. And then, in August, I got a symptom above the neck anyway. In truth, I was relieved to be able to put hope aside.

Most of the things you should worry about come down to water, I had assured Sarah back when the problems with our house were all that woke me up in the morning. Suddenly, though, water itself was waking me up, a few drops tickling my skin at the left-hand corner of my mouth.

'I've started drooling,' I said cheerfully to Sarah one morning, propped up on my elbows in bed and searching for traces of the liquid that I had just felt on my cheek. Sarah found this about as interesting as Leon did – they both headed off to the bathroom to brush their teeth. I lingered for a minute or two. I couldn't find any signs of my dribbling, and it didn't matter anyway. By the time I went to the kitchen for coffee, I had already forgotten what I was looking for.

But the next morning the phantom dribbling had returned. And the morning after. I knew this was extremely bad news, but I also knew that I could not entirely get my head around it at present. Sure, this tiny new symptom was announcing an entire disease: it was confirming that I had MS. Alongside that, though, this new symptom was playful. It was a thing in and of itself.

'Let's not think about it,' I said to Sarah, who surprised me by agreeing. 'Let's just see where it leads.'

This watery tingling sensation indulged me, over the course of a few days, by spreading, from the left corner of my mouth, out along my cheek, down towards the middle of my chin. And it spread upwards too, all the way up the left side of my face to curve in somewhere around my eyebrow.

For a while this was like having a river running down my face, a permanent river that could be felt trickling at all hours. A week or so into it I would continue to search, instinctively, for any sign of actual water, but my hands would always come away dry. The river was clearly cool and subterranean, like the brook made by Hans to aid the adventurers in *Journey to the Centre of the Earth*. Like that river, it seemed to be a benign thing. Not exactly helpful in my case, but still an interesting companion.

Many neurological problems are conspiratorial: it is between me and them, and nobody else can really be admitted. I would be at work, talking on the phone, and there would be water trickling down my face. I would be getting the bus on a dry summer day, water flowing over me and nobody else. I got Leon to touch my face with her tiny fingers on evenings when it was my turn to rock her to sleep; the water would stop for a few seconds and then start to flow again once her hand retracted, continuing to flow as she rolled over and started to snore on the pillow I held her on.

Then, a week after it first started to trickle over my face, the river froze. One day I awoke and the river had ceased to move, transformed into a frosty kind of numbness, tracing the same path down my cheek from my eyebrow to my chin. Occasionally I would get a jolt from it: an icy pulse that ran up the entire side of my face and buried itself above my eye. It caused me to shake or twitch, and then I had to admit to Sarah that the river was still there, albeit in a new form.

'Does it hurt?' she asked one Saturday morning as Leon and I were playing Lego.

'Not really,' I said. 'It's quite nice, really. It's like Christmas.'

'But it's Christmas in your face,' said Sarah.

The obvious conclusion was that the river I had felt was actually a nerve. Like any doomed explorer, I suddenly wanted to map this river and find the source.

It was Leon's birthday, not that she understood that. We could barely understand it ourselves. The scarlet Godzilla who had arrived twelve months ago was now a genial presence in our everyday lives, a smile first thing in the morning when she would awake, a morning picture message if I was working from the office, wearing a saucepan on her head, say, or trying to hug one of the cats. We had decided to celebrate her birthday as a close family, just the three of us. She had loved making marks in a sandpit so much on a recent trip to the park that I had bought her pens and paper as a present. She was fascinated by the pens – the colours, the hard gloss of the plastic – but she was too clumsy to make much practical use of them. Maybe I could use them instead.

I took a piece of paper and started drawing. I was aiming for

a side view of my face, and after a few false starts I had it: a
nerve emerging like a tall, thinly bowed letter *C* on the left of
my face, but with the hint of a protrusion in the middle somewhere, reaching towards my mouth.

I showed this drawing to Sarah, who recognized it immediately. It was the trigeminal nerve, a long stretch of bundled
tissue found on either side of the face, containing both sensory
and motor neurons. It allows you to register a kiss on the cheek.
It allows you to bite and chew. It is quite a nerve.

A bit of googling suggested a name for my underground
river: trigeminal neuralgia. 'There's a society for it,' said Sarah,
turning the computer around to show me the logo, a divided
face, the darker side scarred with a familiar arc of red.

'One of the worst things about getting sick is how many
clubs you can suddenly be a member of,' I said, closing the laptop after scanning a few more links, most of which spoke about
limitless pain and the imperfect surgery options available.
Trigeminal neuralgia, I noted, is occasionally a symptom of
multiple sclerosis.

The limitless pain had never arrived for me, and after a week
or so this frosty nerve started to fade into the background of its
own accord. Not before it caught fire, however: for a couple of
days before the end I marked time by its sudden flare-ups, once
or twice a minute, heat racing over the left side of my face and
also erupting simultaneously in the flesh between the thumb
and first finger of my left hand. Nothing to get excited about.
It was just Christmas, lodged in my face, ablaze.

Still, at times like this, when I am discovering new parts of
the body, I have been tempted to leave the drawing paper
behind and place the wet points of Leon's magic markers
directly on my skin, tracing lines whenever a new nerve ignites,
arcing down over the regular spots: the hands, the cheeks, the
temples, the ridges of my eyebrow, a point next to the big toe

where several nerves converge and the effect is of stepping on spilt droplets of water. Over time, I tell myself, I could photograph these sketches and run them together, creating some kind of living map of hidden paths I have brought to the surface, knowledge I have not earned through study of *Gray's Anatomy* and university classes, but through direct experience. Perhaps this is why patients can seem so irritating to some doctors. We understand so little of the bigger picture but on certain details we are, inevitably, savants.

One night towards the end of August, Sarah and Leon asleep beside me, I sat up late in bed and continued to do what I had spent the last few evenings doing. I was researching multiple sclerosis. Not in a useful way, of course. No chance. I had recently read a single line on a Wikipedia page about the blood-brain barrier and run away from all that, sick at the sheer throbbing thought of it, *the blood-brain barrier*, which I saw as a huge wall of thin sheeting, a cheap shower curtain really, bucking and warping as it struggled to hold back warm, salty tides.

Instead, I approached this research the way I approached everything. Egomaniacally. Selfishly. An investigation into identity. *MS – Celebrities*, rather than *MS – Symptoms*. Who else had this thing that I was about to be given? I sensed again that quiet opportunity to decide: who do I want to be? It's a question that, for me, in my family, surrounded by charismatic grown-ups pitched against one another, always really meant: who do I want to be *like*?

I found a page on Wikipedia: 'List of People with Multiple Sclerosis'. As I scanned down the central column, it occurred to me that I had done this sort of thing before, a long time ago. I hunted for the memory, a tongue darting around after an ulcer. And there it was: back when my parents had divorced. Eleven.

A new school, and the slow dawning that I was the only kid in my class whose parents were not together. I felt special, rather stupidly (reading back through all this I see that I have often felt special, and it has always been stupid), but I was simply the first.

'List of People with Multiple Sclerosis'. The hope, of course, was to find someone I already identified with: someone who was aspirational but within limits, within reach. Jed Bartlet from *The West Wing* was on the list, the character played by Martin Sheen. Of course! I scrolled back through my memories of *The West Wing*, tentatively, in case there was anything to fear, to reject. Bartlet was a genius, a moral rock and a profound yet mercurial thinker. PhD in economics, president of the United States. We did not seem to have much in common.

In fact, Bartlet reminded me of my dad rather than me, and his illness was directed – listlessly, and then with antic bursts – by the needs of the plot anyway. It gave him a mournful gravitas that I suspected I would never grow to assume. One good thing at least: when MS appeared in *The West Wing*, it was always oddly appealing. Bartlet would swoon away in the office. He would bear his suffering nobly on a trip to China and still get the job done.

Bartlet was a bust, in other words, and so were many of the others. I didn't know who Fleur Agema was, although I liked the tumbling music of the name. I had never thought much about Jack Osbourne, beyond the idea that he had always seemed peculiarly huggable. Joan Didion was Bartlet tier, too lofty an ambition for a person who writes about video games, as was Richard Pryor: another genius, another giant.

And Jacqueline du Pré was exactly what I did not want to think about. My sparse mental file on du Pré read: Cut down in her prime? Something bad that made her a monster and then killed her?

Onwards. Iman Ali was not the Iman married to Bowie. Hal Ketchum had another amazing name, but I didn't care about country music. Finally, at the end of a few tense hours, I was left with Teri Garr. Good old ineffectual Teri Garr, the watery, porcelain presence in all those '80s movies I had watched as a kid, the one who was always on the verge of tears because Dustin Hoffman didn't take her seriously in *Tootsie*. She had MS. I did not know this until I saw it on the screen, but I suddenly realized that she already felt like a friend, like an ally.

And Dustin Hoffman was an absolute shit for not taking her seriously. For not taking us seriously.

It was nice to have Teri Garr with me in spirit. I would need her nearby for the next challenge, which was telling my enormous immediate family about what was going on. In my mind this task loomed in front of me with the miserable floodlit tackiness of a regional telethon. An unpopular cause, only third-tier celebrities available for the main event. Phone banks would be required, and we would all draw on the flickering energy of a brittle host, sweating and staring, culled from work on coach tours and cruises, as we drank cold coffee and punched our way through one call after another. The only truly bright spot would be the running total. How many told, how many left to tell. How long now before we can all go home.

As for what to actually say to my family, I had thought about this, and discussed it with Sarah.

'It's probably best to do it once you know for sure,' Sarah said.

'I like the idea of doing it in stages, though,' I argued. 'Bedding it in.'

'Drawing it out?' she said. 'Leading people on?'

'But what about giving them a big shock after the fact?'

Sarah frowned at me. 'It's going to be a big shock however you do it,' she said.

'Exactly,' I said. 'We're agreed, then. Best to do it in stages.'

Up until this point, I had never, in this relationship or any other, ever used the phrase *We're agreed, then*. Thirty-six years of ducking it. And they seemed, in retrospect, like thirty-six very good years.

So, armed with everything but a diagnosis and a practical sense of what MS actually entailed, I got to work. Simon had been a test run, I suppose. It had not been a total disaster. I gave myself a six out of ten on that one. Within twenty minutes or so we had been talking about his daughter and about secondary schools – even if one of us was still secretly talking about the diagnosis.

But if there's one thing I know about test runs, it's this: you just can't have enough of them. So for the second test, I told my boss. It was easy, because I was a coward and I did it over email. My boss was fine about it. He was better than fine. The company would do all they could for me. I appreciated my intense good fortune, and then thought about the individual members of my family. Next up, I needed to try something a little trickier. I turned to Janey.

Janey, my greatest ally in our family, the sibling closest to me in age and temperament. At times, it feels like we have entirely the same brains in our heads, Janey and I, although, clearly, I would now have to stop hoping that this was true.

And let me step back for a moment here. I will not make a habit of this. But it feels useful to admit at this point that I have had an email sitting in my inbox for the last few weeks, sent to me by myself in the dark of night, with no body text and a subject line that simply reads: *What to do with Janey?*

What to do? Because Janey should be everywhere in this book. We are just two years apart and uncommonly close. We live near each other, she married my old boss – they met at my wedding – and she had her first child, Thornton, a few months after Leon was born. For years we were conspirators, as all the best siblings can hope to be at some point. And we were arm-chair anthropologists too, studying with interest the other people in our family and convening, every now and then, to discuss private theories. Many brothers and sisters are close, certainly. Janey and I are so close that nobody else will play board games with us. We are Cluedo close, Monopoly close, able to communicate in what amounts to fragments of code, references long since forged in private. This is the power of shared experience, and I have been told it is odd and uniquely disquieting to hear this stuff in public, when Janey and I are lapping other teams in Articulate, for example, guessing words correctly without appearing to actually say very much to each other.

Over the years I have marvelled at all the small, strange ways in which we are alike, and all the big, delightful ways in which we are different. She is bold, she knows about classics and archaeology. She can read Latin, like my dad, and some-times jokes with him *in Latin*. She doesn't just believe in justice, she is willing to fight for it in public.

And yet what to do with her? Because she is nowhere in this book. She has been nowhere in this illness of mine.

I spoke to her about this the other day. It was over the phone, toddlers in the background on both sides, and I apologized for not having a clearer idea of what to do with her in my narra-tive: no scenes, no killer lines. Not that it's the kind of book where anybody has killer lines.

She said it was her fault. There was the birth of Thornton, and the cocoon of early motherhood, but there was also an unwillingness to engage with what was happening – what it meant for me, and what it meant for the rest of us.

I believe that she believes that. But I do not believe that. I think that I have kept her away, not out of some misguided kindness, but out of a dark sense of self-preservation. I could not confront what I would see reflected in Janey. I did not want to see our minds begin to diverge.

So. Let me just say this: my sister and I, we went through everything in our childhood together. She has a long frame and flat feet that make her look like she is stomping everywhere she walks. She is kind and patient and fiercely, wonderfully, unpredictable. The radio in her house is always tuned to Radio 3, which inspires a kind of middle-class awe in me even now. And she will not let the important things go, not ever — and what more, really, can you say for somebody?

And yet, I used her when I told her about MS. The kindest way to frame this — by which I mean, of course, the way that is kindest to me — is to say that I was so secure in my friendship with Janey that I felt I could abuse it a little. I could hone my powers of manipulation on her to better tackle the bigger, trickier problems in my family and the question of how to break bad news to them quickly, painlessly, efficiently and effectively.

I approached the Janey problem by thinking: What would work on me? I decided it was best to get her on board, to give her a way of being helpful — a knot to worry at in private. I met her after work in the coffee shop inside Jubilee Library in Brighton. The coffee is fine here, but the view is wonderful: look out through the huge glass windows and Jubilee Square is filled with nutty Brighton life. Look up, and the entire reference section hovers above you, a floor that rests on spindly stilts, lit by three huge light wells in the roof. It is the perfect place to lend a little atmosphere to even the most mundane of conversations, and when the conversation isn't mundane, the bustle and wide-open spaces of the library seem to work against themselves to create a kind of intimacy.

We would need intimacy. I explained that something was possibly wrong and a neurologist had suggested multiple sclerosis. But it didn't seem likely. Still, I was going to have to tell everyone else in the family about this, and would she be willing to help me smooth things over if and when it turned out to be a false alarm?

Only thinking over all this now do I appreciate just what a horrible liar I am. I was robbing Janey of a chance to have an emotional response. I pushed her past the moment of revelation and landed her, temporarily, in a moment that I already knew would never come, a moment when it had all turned out to be a big nothing. I knew, fully knew, that I would then be able to move past that false outcome to the next *real* moment – the it's-all-true-after-all moment – and I still wouldn't have had to deal with the actual instance of revelation. I would have hopped past it. I would have outplayed it.

So I was turning Janey into my pawn. I was using her. I know now that when you tell someone that something bad is happening to you, you have to remember that this is a moment for them as well as a moment for you. You have responsibilities to get them through it, and to get them through it honestly.

To bewilder Janey even further – and to give me an easy exit to the bus and then home, I had Garr saved up for the inevitable question: What is multiple sclerosis anyway? *I don't know, Janey, but remember Teri Garr from* Tootsie? *She has it. She was Phoebe's mother in* Friends*, so she must be fine.* (Yes, incidentally, she was Phoebe's mother. But watch her in *Friends*. Watch, in many of the scenes she's in, how little she actually *moves*. Watch the force, the deftly concealed force, with which she grips the nearby furniture. A pro.)

I got through another sister and a brother like that. Saz, the youngest and most direct of the Donlans, no match at all for my skilful dishonesty. Paul, the eldest and most distant. Saz sounded glum but hopeful. Paul sounded like a hard man in *EastEnders*. 'I can't say I'm happy about it,' he said, as if I had announced I was foreclosing on his launderette. 'But okay.' They both asked what MS meant, and in both cases I realized afresh that I didn't really know. I realized too how inadequate I was as a sibling. My last few communications with Paul and Saz had been the following: *I'm getting married, will you come to the wedding? I'm having a baby, will you come to visit?* Now this.

Ben and Mum were both difficult. Mum was unreadably vague, asking, in a tranquillized way, if MS was what Stephen Hawking had. 'No,' I said. 'It's what Teri Garr has.'

'Oh, *Young Frankenstein*,' she replied. That was enough for her: no questions, which I interpreted, foolishly, as disinterest rather than swiftly pooling fright.

Ben was a call that I had been truly dreading, so I kept it short. He offered advice. 'They'll give you three things it could be, they always do,' he said. 'Two won't be scary. The last one will. And the thing you have will be the last one and they'll already know it.'

I cast my mind back to what Quill had said. Three things it could be. And the last one?

Dad was the final call. Dad, who had been so brilliant with Ben. Dad, who had responded to drama by taking control, by becoming an expert. I had saved him until last because it would be like coming home again.

And I knew it would be like coming home for a simple reason. Dad does this stuff all the time. It was his job for thirty-odd years, dealing with disorders and diagnoses. It was part of the reason he got on so well with Sarah from the start – a deep fascination with things that go wrong with people's heads. But actually, now I think of it, is fascination the right word?

For many years, my dad's job was a little like Quill's: observation and evaluation. He would meet clients, and he would have a few minutes to watch them and decide what might be going on inside their minds.

Social work was a distressing business, and my dad has always been a sensitive man. Faced with the daily horrors of his job (and going home each night to a house full of young children) I sometimes wonder if his expertise, his expansive knowledge of psychological syndromes and neurological deficits, became a form of protection. I don't think he ever reduced his cases to the point where they were intellectual puzzles to solve, but there may have been a cushion provided by the process of assessment.

He was successful working like this, I think, but it had knock-on effects. Over the years, Dad became very used to studying people.

And at times he has struggled to stop doing it. As long as I have known him, Dad has been a people watcher. (Many Donlans are. My grandmother liked nothing more than sitting by the window and scrutinizing anybody who went past. She even had a term for it: *gentling*.) But Dad is also a people diagnoser. He cannot walk through a crowd without noting the tics and quirks around him. He cannot stop finding what he has taught himself to look for.

(Social work also fostered a flair for inappropriate conversation. I once brought a new girlfriend round for dinner when something over dessert caused Dad to explain at great length Freud's theory of childhood sexuality.)

Awkward as all this could be, it has flowed from the stuff I love about him. Dad has devoted himself to helping others. And, through this, he has broken a wretched cycle, as the gentle son of a bad father who was himself raised by a bad father.

So no, I was not too worried about Dad. I knew he could handle it.

And inevitably he couldn't handle it at all.

'Dad,' I said over the phone one evening, Leon sitting in my lap, facing away from me, rubbing her fuzzy blonde head under my chin, 'there's something wrong with my hands.'

'Arthritis?' he asked almost instantly. 'Your Aunt Luanne had it.'

I thought: My Aunt Luanne had been a massive boozer, more like. Northern California, married to the local sheriff, she once shot her TV set because she thought it was an intruder.

But I would not be distracted. 'Something else,' I said.

'Familial tremor?' asked Dad. 'A shaking in your right hand? All the men in our family have it.'

Christ, Dad, is this how you treated your clients? The next five minutes unspooled like this, as Dad tried to stave off my specifics by countering with specifics of his own, controlling the diagnosis or at least delaying it, burying it among possibilities and anecdotes. And he had a lot of anecdotes. Did I know I had a great-aunt of some kind who had become mentally incapable after being scared by a horse? Or was she kicked by a horse, with the same result? No matter either way. Or it could be a trapped nerve. It could be a problem with my foot – sounds weird, but it does happen! Uncle Marty –

'The doctor thinks it might be multiple sclerosis,' I said eventually, cutting in.

The line crackled. I said nothing more.

'Multiple sclerosis.' Dad exhaled.

I closed my eyes and saw him easing back in his desk chair, trying to fit this idea into his life. I felt Leon's hair rubbing against my chin, her skull warm and fragile.

'Like Bartlet?' he asked.

'Like Teri Garr,' I said, purely out of spite. 'Bartlet's not real.'

Dad thought for a few seconds more. 'It doesn't run in the family,' he said, and fell silent again. Maybe he was running through all the cases he had ever dealt with in social work, pulling the mug shots. Maybe part of him was preparing to slip my own photo in there with them.

'Did you deal with any MS in your work?' I asked at last.

'Once or twice,' said Dad, reluctant to continue. I forced him on with silence.

'I remember one thing,' he said. 'A paper I read that I'll try to dig out.' The thought of digging something out seemed to lend him energy in this difficult moment. 'There's this theory of MS personality,' he continued. 'The idea is that people develop a way of blaming other people for the illness – they externalize it by brutalizing people around them. It's a personality change. The pain, the confusion, chips away at you and you become cruel.'

I thought about how I had just treated Janey – but that was just me being me, sadly. 'Thanks, Dad,' I said. 'I'll look out for that.'

In the run-up to diagnosis, I was diagnosed many times. I imagined it again and again, the way that some people imagine their wedding day, perhaps, or the day they graduate, or the birth of their children. I would awake from a dream of diagnosis and have a daydream diagnosis before getting up. I tried different reactions. *What does this mean for me?* I might ask if I was feeling bold. *How many years do I have, how many good years?*

I knew my own diagnosis was looming. It would be making its way to me, but how? For endless summer days, I was expecting a letter, an email, a phone call. Maybe Quill would ring me at work, and I would have to duck into a side office and be told what we both already suspected. Maybe his secretary would reach me on the bus and I would have two agonies – the agony of waiting to call her back from somewhere private, and the agony of then waiting for the meeting she was calling to arrange.

Yet, all the time I waited for this call, I was getting calls every hour anyway. That summer, Carphone Warehouse had decided that I was due an upgrade, and even though I promised them I really wasn't, I had to answer the phone every time it rang, because it appeared on my screen as a scary unlisted number. Each time this happened, I had to get into character: I had to assume the role of the doomed hero in the pivotal scene in a movie. And then ten seconds later I had to work out which facial expression I had assumed in order to switch it when I was suddenly confronted with Carl or Ian or Jess just asking if I'd thought of moving to Android now that my contract was up. And did I want any bolt-ons?

It was maddening, but it was also a great gift from Carphone Warehouse — and I'm not talking about bolt-ons here. I was longing to take myself seriously in this moment above all others, and I discovered again and again that I just couldn't. The world was playing this as comedy.

And then euphoria.

The fifth of September 2014. My daughter took her first steps on the day I was diagnosed — a juxtaposition so perfect, so trite, so filled with the tacky artifice of real life that I am generally too embarrassed to tell anybody about it. I still watch the film of this moment — it's actually the film of her second attempt because I refused, righteously, to watch the first through the lens of my phone. It is early evening, after Sarah and I have returned from the hospital. Leon is standing by the coffee table in the lounge, able to hold herself up on her legs as long as she is gripping something. Then an idea comes to her, and she decides to pursue it. Frowning, she lurches forward, knees bent and spread, arms at her sides as rigid as a Frankenstein or a

Dracula doing the werewolf dance from 'Thriller'. One foot jolts in front of the other and she is crossing the room, and it dawns on her: this is walking. She reaches me, palms flat and smacking against my legs, and then she collapses in laughter. I'm laughing too. I turn off the camera and yet I can remember what I said to Sarah as we both beamed at each other. 'Today was a good day.'

And it was, even before Leon walked. No phone calls were involved; the letter from Quill booking an appointment had finally come a week beforehand, and Sarah was with me in the afternoon when I descended into the neurology ward once more. It felt weird to take this journey with Sarah, so I flattened it into an inane tour. That room, I remember my brother in there with a line in his head. I remember this used to be a waiting room, and I sat here with Dad while Ben had his surgery. There was a local news programme on that evening: dinner ladies who wore fairy costumes as they served the kids. Dad and I had been up so long we started to laugh helplessly at the sight of them.

Quill was waiting for us in an office next to a murky fish tank. Reversal, inversion: I had been feeling pretty good, physically, for the last few weeks, my symptoms reduced to tingling fingers and not much else. Quill looked absolutely wrecked, grey skin, dark shadows under his eyes, and a long queue of patients outside.

He was direct. I can't remember the words he used, but I remember that he was formal about it, and I remember that I found that obscurely touching – perhaps because of the firm friendship between the two of us that had been established, by this point, entirely in my own mind. I gripped Sarah's hand and Quill told me that I had multiple sclerosis. Relapsing-remitting multiple sclerosis. No need for a second opinion: it was a classic case.

I thought I was prepared for this. But I must not have been. Because as Quill spoke, I felt relief. A huge, warm rush of it. Relief that I knew for certain, of course. But also relief that a hundred little fears I had not allowed myself to voice had gone unmet. Motor neurone disease – could that start with tingling? (No.) Parkinson's – that *does* start with tingling, right? (No.) Even MS itself could be far worse than I had thought. Primary-progressive. Secondary-progressive – maybe I had been so absent in terms of the day-to-day business of my own life that I had actually missed the entire period of relapsing and remitting and landed straight in the advanced form.

I sank back in my seat and leaned against Sarah.

Pity neurologists. Pity them. People say the strangest things to neurologists. They say: My hands feel like they're getting bigger. They say: I feel like I've got three legs. I once said to one of my neurologists: 'I woke up in the night and my eye, my left eye, was slipping down my face, and I've spent the last week with my head tilted to the right to even everything out.' People say all this, and then, even worse, they never listen to the response. 'No patient really listens to a diagnosis,' a neurologist told me recently, pondering, aloud, how to improve his own performance of this difficult task. 'They hear the first sentence, and then they're gone.'

The rest is a blur. Quill explained MS to us both. He explained that symptoms vary, and can be spread across a wide range of the body's territories. He talked about the various types of MS and countered my enthusiasm for relapsing-remitting slightly by stating that while I had the best type to get, I had the worst kind of the best type.

'Your scans are dramatic,' he said. 'You have relapsing-remitting, but it seems to be highly active.'

Perversely, this was possibly also good news – of a kind, at least. It meant that I instantly met the requirements for treatment.

And through all this, I was, of course, not really listening. I was thinking: I can handle this. This sounds like something I can deal with. And I was leaning against Sarah, feeling the rise and fall of her breathing as she listened for us.

And I was also thinking, of all things, about a movie Sarah and I had recently watched: a documentary about Ferran Adrià, the greatest chef in the world, a man from Catalonia who spent half a year constructing a menu of tart, contradictory delights to serve during the other half, in a restaurant that had a waiting list measured out in decades until he eventually shuttered the place on a whim. I thought of the food, which lay scattered, spiralled and arched on the plate, heavy with glossy droplets. All the food looked like something alien and unknowable, and then the taste provided a rush of conflicting certainties. The whole thing was a dance of context, context removed and context replaced, context exploded. Each bite must be dizzying, a diagnosis, a tidal-wave return of certainty. This is the power of context restored, the astonishing power of suddenly knowing exactly where you are and what you have been doing all along.

Quill walked us to the door. I suddenly worried that I was never going to see this man again. This man who had diagnosed me, who had brought my world to some kind of order. 'I need to ask,' I said. 'Are you going to stick with me? Are you my guy?'

Americanisms will never come easy to a man like Quill. He is too much of a witness to assume the role of the protagonist that American language requires. Still, he was game. 'I'm your guy,' he laughed.

'I can't tell you what that means to me,' I said to him, and I held out my hand like the bad soap actor I was.

He took it and then – I will never forget this – he put his other hand on the other side of mine too. I stared into his tired eyes and now I started to cry.

On my way out, I said to Sarah, 'He's amazing, isn't he? He's amazing. Like that chef!' I could not explain myself to her, but she knew what I meant. With great delicacy and kindness, Quill had taken me from one world and led me into another.

Suddenly, there was no time left to me.

I hadn't planned much so far, but I had planned this: I knew exactly what I wanted to do in the days and perhaps weeks following my diagnosis. I would go to bed for about a fortnight, luxuriating in the warmth of some self-prescribed compassionate leave from work. Then I would flop around the house in a dressing gown, bony arm flung across my face, and maybe I would quote T. S. Eliot out loud until someone noticed how resolute I was being about all of this. I had mini tours planned, of the kind Tony Blair executed when he left power: travelling the country to see the spots that had made me who I am, perhaps. I imagined late-night calls to distant university friends and the odd old girlfriend, all of whom would be delighted to hear from me because I had news from, if not quite the other side, then some grey no man's land of barbed experience that was proximate to it.

None of this happened. September was a rattling blur of Facebook messages from old colleagues, meetings at work to see if I had the right chair for my needs, cards in the post and newspaper clippings, often from the *Mail*, that pretended to offer miracle cures but were really eight columns of wallowing in the horror of losing your mind and your body, with a cheery *deus ex machina* at the end, provided by an extra cup of coffee each morning, or by drinking hot water that had been graced with the fleeting presence of a lemon. I kept all these clippings. I even read some of them. Wretched as they are, they are also dear to me, because they represent what people wish they could do for you when they know they can do nothing: they wish they could cure you.

Leon ate all of October whole, and it was a gorgeous sight. She had chosen this strange, post-diagnosis vacuum to stage one of her mad cognitive eruptions, of which walking, working that arms-spread, knees-locked, Monster-Mash stagger across the living room on the day of my meeting with Quill, was just the first seismic rumble. Words were bubbling out of her now, proto-sentences announcing strange ambitions and desires. Her mind seemed too big for her head.

And then there was my illness. Not the symptomatic side, which had conveniently died away, leaving me feeling like a fraud as I explained my tragedy to neighbours on the green and tried to unpick the semantic space for them — and for myself — between an incurable disease and a fatal one. Instead, I was suddenly dealing with the upswing, the return volley, the counterforce: now I had something official to treat, there could be treatment plans.

This sounds like a positive development, and it was. But it didn't always feel like that. Years ago, before Leon was born, I sat in a restaurant with a friend of mine and, surrounded by his two kids, who were running about and driving tiny die-cast cars over the tops of the tables, the underneaths of the tables, over their forearms and elbows and knees, I asked what it was like. What was parenthood like when it was exploding all around you? My friend grew serious and apparently started to channel some forgotten 1980s power ballad: he explained that the highs were very high and the lows were very low. But that's not the defining trait, he said. The defining trait is that the highs and the lows are pushed together so tightly that you can't tell the difference. You can't catalogue what happens in any way; you just have to experience it in an endless rush, and react as appropriately as you are able to.

The race towards treatment plans was a bit like this. The highs were high, the lows were low, and I struggle to separate the two even now.

The facts are simple. If you have primary-progressive MS, in which symptoms emerge over time and with no respite, there are no treatments available. For over a century, it was the same for relapsing-remitting. But in the last thirty years, this has changed, as a range of new therapies have come online. The rate of development is dazzling. When I was experiencing my first symptoms of relapsing-remitting MS, there were eight therapies available. By the time I was asked to make my choice, there were ten. I am extremely grateful.

But that is where the simple stuff ends.

It is early autumn. I am reading a letter from Quill. While he remains my neurologist, he explains, he is not a specialist in MS, and so he is bringing in a specialist to look after me for the foreseeable future. He has also arranged for me to see an MS nurse regularly. I am not keen on the idea of having a nurse – not at thirty-six.

No time to think of that. I am sitting opposite the MS specialist. My new neurologist. Dr Koenig. She is softly spoken and clearly brilliant, explaining to me that the piece of paper I am holding, which lists the ten available therapies, does not really list ten in my case, because my MS is probably too powerful for many of them. There are two viable candidates for now: a pill that is extremely effective at cutting the rate of relapses, but often poorly tolerated, and an infusion that is even better, in her opinion.

I am trying to ask about some of the scary side effects of the infusion that I have read about, and she is trying to explain that the side effects are rare, relatively speaking, and that they will do a blood test to clarify further the specific risks in my case. Mainly, though, we are both being interrupted by my dad. I have brought him along to this because I know how brilliant he was with Ben. He became an expert so quickly. I want him here to make notes, because I know that I will not be able to remember everything Dr Koenig tells me. Sadly, it turns out my dad cannot make notes in a gentle manner. It looks, I realize with growing nausea, like he is here to invigilate, to monitor Dr Koenig's performance. Partway through a crucial discussion regarding what characterizes a relapse in the first place, Dad announces that his pen has stopped working. Does Dr Koenig have one to lend him?

She is unfazed by this, of course. She works among the sick and the incurable, so managing social awkwardness is pretty basic stuff. She treats us far more graciously than we deserve, and as I head for the door, struggling to accept the scale of the decision that faces me, she stops me and says: 'You will never be alone in this.' I still cannot think of an adequate response to that.

It is November. I am looking at that piece of paper with all but two of the treatments crossed off, and now I am climbing stairs, three flights of them, to visit Jennifer, my new MS nurse. I do not want to visit Jennifer, which is why it has taken me until the brink of November to make the journey. I have deleted emails. I have stuffed letters in drawers half-read.

I worry that Jennifer is going to make me sick. I don't know why I worry about this. Maybe because she is a nurse, and if you have a nurse you must be in a pretty bad way. Maybe because she works all day with other MS patients, and I worry, secretly, shamefully, that they will make clear the trajectory that I am now on. Already I have decided something: I have decided that I do not really want to meet anybody else who has MS if I can avoid it. I am suddenly scared of other people with MS and the glimpse of the possible future they provide. I know this is foolish, selfish, short-sighted and cruel. I know that it is shameful, but still, I want to tell Jennifer straight off: do not make me join a group of any kind.

I should not have worried. Jennifer is a tiny American with curly hair and an exquisite calm to her. Her very presence suggests that everything going on outside the door has just stopped for a few moments, and we should take some time to worry only about what is going on right now. I remember little of our first meeting, which is mainly form-filling and arranging future meetings at three-month intervals. What I do remember, though, is that we sit in an office that Jennifer makes airy and cheerful despite the fact that there are no windows and the only decorative item in the room is a model of a human femur, split down the middle to reveal the textured pink bone marrow within.

Before I go, I tell Jennifer that she should know upfront that I don't know what I'm doing – I think I mean in this disease, but also, possibly, in life – and that I hope this is okay. She shakes my hand briskly and tells me something extraordinary. She tells me that my disease is unprecedented. That everyone's MS is. 'You will become the only expert there will ever be in your illness,' she says. And I believe it. I creaked up the three flights to meet Jennifer. I practically skip down them. What she has told me sounds like the preparation for an adventure.

And then, finally, I am in another room, in another local hospital, and I am facing two infusion nurses who are here to learn of my treatment decisions: which of the two miracle drugs – my description, not anybody else's – have I decided to take?

As I remember this meeting, and as I described it to my dad afterwards, I was extremely eloquent and calm. I explained that this decision was impossibly difficult, harder even than my diagnosis, and that this was because inside the dawning realization that something was wrong with me, inside the nested realization that certain things would never be right again, here was something I could actually do about it. A decision. And that decision was terrifying. How strange: I was happy to be knocked about by fate. I was used to it. But now, after making this decision, I could no longer be blameless. Everyone had explained that the treatment plan was ultimately up to me, and although I had pretty much begged everyone to make this decision for me anyway, everyone had, infuriatingly, stayed true to their word.

Of course I blamed the people who would not make the decision on my behalf: Sarah, my dad, Leon perhaps, as I rocked her on her pillow each night, as hot air seemed to pulse between my ears, my eyeballs itchy and scorched. This was not MS I was experiencing: this was the endless migraine of angry indecision.

Still, to live with all that and still be so eloquent, I told Dad afterwards. Not bad, I concluded.

Except my memory is wrong. None of this happened the way I remember it.

'You were so sweary that day,' Sarah said to me recently. 'It was "fucking this, fucking that". It was, "I'm not fucking taking these drugs."'

'Was I really?' I wanted to ask, but I knew that she was right.

And maybe, if I really put the work in, I can remember the swearing after all. Those fucking drugs.

It was the side effects I could not get past. The best drug available had these extremely rare side effects, and I knew I could not live with that kind of worry.

I should have taken that drug. I knew that then and I know it now. I also know that I could never have taken it, because good as it is and as unlikely as the truly awful side effects were, I could not have lived with the side effect that would have definitely turned up – the side effect that involved lying in bed every night imagining fluids building up over time, imagining pipes bursting and buckets overflowing, imagining all the dark, irreversible things that a life-saving serum might be doing inside me. Instead, I rejected medicine. I rejected this whole choice that had been flung at me. I told the infusion nurses I wasn't going to take either of the drugs.

And then, just as quickly, I understood that I was going to make a choice after all.

I would love to say that it was the thought of Leon or of Sarah or Ben that won me around. But it was something I saw in the eyes of one of the nurses, both of whom had that classic NHS bearing: compassion tempered with steel. What I saw was a sense that I didn't realize how good I had it, that after centuries of MS ravaging people, unstitching them day by day with no hope of treatment at all, I was alive in the first twenty years in which there was anything at all that could be done for someone like me. Twenty years ago there was no treatment. Now there were ten. They were all imperfect, of course, and none of them would cure me, but they were something. And I had to choose *something*.

I also understood that I had travelled further than I could have imagined already. I had become Ben at last: so angry that I wouldn't countenance my options. Now it was not so huge a leap to travel past that and make a choice of my own, even if it was the wrong choice. The wrong choice, yes, but not the wrongest possible choice. So I chose the pill.

And then things slowed down. We had another quiet Christmas, just the three of us, as the days dwindled away to nothing and the sea on the coast road turned as grey as a piece of slate. On a cold white morning in January, the wind roaring outside, I sat down in an armchair and pressed that morning's pill out of its packaging, where it sat next to a little image of the sun. The evening's pill, sat next to an image of the moon, awaited me, and every day and every night for the foreseeable there would be suns and moons and pills to go with them.

I swallowed the pill and gripped the edges of my chair, like a time traveller in a movie, about to be hurtled through g-forces and into the unknown. An hour later, bouncing Leon around on my knee, I felt it, a hot prickling at my temples that spread to my cheeks and nose. 'I'm having a hot flush,' I said to Sarah, laughing at the painful pleasure of it. 'I read about these. It's working. It's working.'

The First Recorded Case of MS

MS was first described in the 1860s, and it is sometimes viewed as a nineteenth-century disease: a disease of cities and factories, pollution and poor living conditions. Some neurologists argue, however, that the nineteenth century was merely the right time for MS to be identified, since industrialization meant that medicine was also going through its own period of rapid transformation.

And every now and then someone uncovers a historical case that could point to the appearance of MS before the nineteenth century. It is enduringly hard to make a judgement, partly because the historical record is not filled with detailed descriptions of neurological patients and their individual ailments, and partly because MS's vast constellation of possible symptoms can make the disease tricky to diagnose even now.

Of these early cases, two tend to stand out. In the twelfth century, a young Icelandic woman named Halldora grew weak in the limbs and gradually lost the ability to walk. For three years she was bedridden. She saw only slight improvements in her condition until Thorlak Thorhallsson, a famed religious healer who would become the patron saint of Iceland, appeared in a friend's dream and urged Halldora to go on a pilgrimage – a pilgrimage that, once undertaken on a stretcher, eventually cured her.

Halldora was far from Thorlak's only success story. And, reading through some of his other notable victories, as described in 'The Saga of Bishop Thorlak', it's hard to be inspired by the overall quality of the contemporary reporting. Women were cured of devilry by drinking oil Thorlak had consecrated. A small cow that fell from a cliff and was 'completely smashed up' was reassembled instantly by his intervention. He calmed seas and extinguished blazes. A number of people walked again following his involvement. Is Halldora's narrative reliable enough, or even detailed enough, to suggest MS had appeared in the twelfth century?

St Lidwina of Schiedam's narrative benefits from better documentation. A Dutch mystic living in the late fourteenth and early fifteenth centuries, Lidwina led a healthy life until she broke a rib in a fall while ice skating at the age of sixteen. An abscess formed, slowing her recovery, and she continued to have difficulty walking long after her injury had healed.

Over the next few years, she developed headaches and shooting pains in her teeth. By nineteen, she had sporadic pain throughout her whole body. She was still unable to walk without assistance, had weakness in her right arm and was also blind in her right eye. Later in life, she saw angels and spoke with God. These instances were sometimes accompanied by periods in which the severity of her ailments was reduced.

Lidwina is still not a natural fit for an MS patient. Descriptions of her illness include some strange details. Blood poured from her mouth, ears and nose. She shed skin, bones and parts of her intestines. Her bodily odour was sweet-smelling and sometimes cured the sick.

Still, in among the offal and the holy miracles, there is something that definitely sounds a little like MS here: a disease of blindness and paralysis and pain, with a form that means the worst of it comes and goes. I can easily imagine Lidwina, fearful of what was happening to her, and, like all patients in all eras, casting around for the answer that most lined up with the thinking of the time.

Regardless, for the first verifiable case of MS you have to look to the nineteenth century.

In December 1822, Augustus d'Este, a grandson of George III, travelled from Ramsgate to the Highlands to visit a close friend and discovered, upon arriving, that his friend had died. 'There being so many persons present I struggled violently not to weep,' he wrote after the funeral, noting endearingly that his struggles were unsuccessful.

In the days that followed all this weeping, the world was changed – viewed as if through tears. But d'Este was no longer weeping. He noted in his diary that his eyes were 'attacked', and he was relieved when the situation resolved itself as quickly as it had appeared. He may have thought, at the time, that this would be the end of it. But in truth it was the beginning.

Reading back over the records d'Este kept throughout his life – he was twenty-eight at the time of his first symptoms, and he died in 1848 at the age of fifty-four – he was an exemplary patient, endlessly optimistic, and keenly alert to any change in his physical being.

Still, it is a spooky experience to read through a litany of familiar symptoms, understanding that this is the first time they had been recorded in such detail. In 1825, Augustus has spots in front of his eyes. In 1826, his blurred vision returns, while diplopia, or double vision, follows a year later during a scorching trip to Lausanne. This time, it is accompanied by 'a torpor or indistinctness of feeling about the Temple of my left eye'. A torpor or indistinctness of feeling. At times, it feels like MS is getting its first poet as well as its first patient.

And it continues. His strength leaves him for a period of a few days. He suffers numbness and a loss of sensation. He collapses. He has fatigue and impotence. His bowels are good and then his bowels are very bad: 'a most unsatisfactory state'. He has balance problems and spasms – particularly in the morning upon waking.

Throughout all of this, a secondary narrative slowly emerges, as he is subjected to strange contemporary treatments by a shuffled array of doctors. He is blooded by leeches. He is made to drink and bathe in 'Steel-water'. Another doctor prescribes beefsteaks, twice a day, as well as London porter, sherry and Madeira. (In ancient Egypt the doctors were priests; by the nineteenth century in Europe, they are often chefs.) D'Este's legs are rubbed with brushes and his back is rubbed with liniment. He slaps himself in the groin to bring his strength back temporarily. He undergoes, in his later years, a 'course of Electricity'.

And this is all from the doctors who try to help him. Another says that there is nothing wrong with him. This doctor says that he has seen worse.

Throughout all this, d'Este's behaviour is glorious. He seems cheerful until the end, despite his increasing reliance upon 'a chair with wheels'. His notes capture not only the symptoms of his illness, but many incidental details that provide crucial context – the heat of Lausanne, for example, where he first encountered diplopia.

And this is perhaps the thing I find most noble about d'Este: he never stops trying to put his experience into words, even when there are no words available any more, and even when, unable to write legibly, someone else has to make notes on his behalf.

We should remember Augustus d'Este for his passions, for the things that clearly moved him: for enlightenment, for his support of aboriginal peoples, for his belief that native Americans should have titles to their lands.

Instead, history remembers him for his illness and the great delicacy with which he drew out its various elements. 'I know not how to give an idea of it,' he writes one day towards the end. And this remains a central problem of neurology – at least from a patient's perspective.

5. The Dead Teach the Living

I follow a pathologist on Instagram. She is from New Jersey, and covered in tattoos. Roses cluster around her neck; vines and butterflies wind through radioactive clouds as they race across her shoulders. Her name is Mrs Angemi, and her motto is *mortui vivos docent* : the dead teach the living.

Mrs Angemi's feed is an explosion of human suffering. Flesh is stripped from hands and arms (they call it de-gloving). Gunshot wounds knock ragged holes in skulls. Cancer spins crazed shapes out of a glossy red colon, out of a blackened lung.

And interspersed with these images are pictures of her children on day trips, or plugs for her T-shirts, including one in which the dura mater (literally 'tough mother'; a protective layer that lies just under the skull) is peeled back to expose the brain.

Strange things happen when Mrs Angemi gets mixed in with the rest of my Instagram feed. It's meatballs and chopped daikon and then, 'This is what a leg amputation looks like!' Velázquez at the Prado, take-out coffee from Mexico, followed by a scrubbed hand delicately holding the tiny brain of a foetus, smooth and cream-coloured like a seared scallop.

Mrs Angemi's mission seems beautiful to me. She wants to share the truth about the human body, to offer bright views of our hidden worlds – and she wants to do this on Instagram of all places. She shoves death in the midst of life – in the midst of this artifice of life. She trusts death to earn its place as one spectacle among others.

I tried to explain the appeal of this to my dad once, and he raised an eyebrow and said nothing, reacting in the same way he had, many years ago, when Ben announced that he wanted to paint his bedroom black, even though it was also my bedroom. (Ben was argued down to a deep Rothko red, which was actually even more oppressive.)

'Is this an MS thing?' Dad asked eventually.

'It's not,' I said. 'At least, I don't think it is.'

Mrs Angemi doesn't do MS. I suspect that the disease is simply not dramatic enough. The plaques or scars that MS leaves in the brain will not make a good enough picture without the stage management of an MRI, and there are other feeds for MRIs on Instagram. Still, I think about her work every day. I think about the story that plays out in her photographs, regardless of disease or injury. Stitching, bruising, the inevitable ravages. This is not always death. This is often just what being alive looks like.

And Dad was wrong, even if, looking back, I realize he didn't actually put his judgement into words. Seeing this endless stream of images is not maudlin. It fills me with a dizzying rush of life. I open the browser, draw a deep breath, prepare myself for the worst, and then I load up Mrs Angemi's page and study what she has posted that day. I look for about five seconds. And then I breathe out, close my eyes and feel incredibly aware of my own existence, of the absolute limits of my own body. I feel my heart beating. I feel my hands tingling and sparking. I feel a roaring in my ears that seems to be life itself pushing onwards one moment at a time. It is an amazing thing: the high-altitude giddiness of having survived an encounter with something so vivid. Proof of life.

I felt this same thrill – this same woozying throb of freshly achieved clarity – in the days just after my diagnosis. Sure, I experienced an enormous upsurge of smugness, a sense of being granted privileged information of some kind, information that I should not share with others even if I could. But I also felt more worthwhile things. Again and again I came back to that thought: *the dead teach the living*. I compared the head rush of that Instagram feed with the head rush of diagnosis, and I wondered if, maybe, we are most alive in the presence of illness.

And then one day this thought led me back to Gene.

My mother, who believes in ghosts, who believes in God, has received only one message from the other side. It was the early 1990s, and it was a message from someone she knew, her own recently dead mother, who had been a bland kind of tyrant, dour and cold as a frozen outdoor tap. Her mother had left her much, if you were counting a fondness for robins and a thick layer of emotional scarring. In the material realm, she'd also left her a book of English poems, the spine frayed and the cloth cover made waxy through handling. One day my mother opened this book to discover that her mother had marked poems for her to read – poems picked out with precise slashes of a sharp pencil. This one. This one.

This one:

> Remember me when I am gone away,
> Gone far away into the silent land . . .

As if she would be allowed to forget. What these messages said, once decoded – and it was not a tough one to crack – was: *Me. It is all still about me – or at least it should be, if you are doing it right.*

Gene also returned to me through a book, but the message was, typically, far gentler. One night in early January I found myself lingering in the bath with a novel I had not read in years: *3001: The Final Odyssey*, by Arthur C. Clarke. The story begins with a dead man returning after many centuries away. Frank Poole of *2001*, knocked into space by HAL, orbiting through the ice in the lonely darkness beyond Jupiter, is caught and defrosted in the distant future. Somewhere in the early chapters I decided to break off, marking my page with a post-card, and check the endpapers, where I had once taken to writing the date a book was first read. (It costs nothing to write the date in the front pages of a book the first time you read it, and yet it is a sweet gift, a priceless jolt of reverie when, years later, you open the cover and think: Oh, yes.)

2000. A giddy, year-long spell at Sussex University. The MA I got at the end of it mentioned literature and visual culture, but Sussex had been so bracingly interdisciplinary I had quickly lost my way and ended up spending most of the course reading about postmodern anthropology. This is even stupider than it sounds, really: it means I was excited about understanding the social structures of people who cannot agree about reality in the first place. 'Nice work,' Mum had said to me when I told her what I had been up to. 'That will come in useful when you're looking for a job.' But it did, I guess: I now write about video games.

And the course was only half the fun anyway. Brighton! I experienced a sudden shock of brisk imagery: riding the Falmer train on a sharp-aired Thursday morning, heading over the viaduct with its golden glimpse of a cold, sunlit avenue leading to the distant sea; walking head down across Library Square as the first huge wet fragments of snow started to fall in December; waking in one of those sagging chairs by the photocopy centre to hear the last call that the building was being locked for the evening. At any one of those points I could imagine the book in my bag or tucked under an arm, cover jacket removed so people might assume it was Derrida or *The Mass Ornament*.

And then I looked at the postcard I was using as a bookmark.

The postcard was clearly an artefact, edges thick and fuzzy with time, the white of its message face turning a sour yellow. And that handwriting. I felt almost dizzy as the words came into focus. I flipped the card over: Boston, the English one. And on the back. 'I'm in Boston, the English one, seeing a bit of the world . . .' I looked at the addressee: 'Chris Donlan, Sussex University. History Dept (?).' Good guess, but wrong. And with it a memory of reaching into my cubbyhole in the common room one day, expecting unwelcome essay feedback and finding: this. A postcard trailing a warm sense of the man who wrote it. That shrewd, slightly hamsterish face, that warm, edgeless voice. Gene had returned to me, like Frank Poole. Just as vivid, just as unexpected, just as welcome. And from, it seemed, a similar distance.

Can you speak to the dead? The truth, I think, is that it is easy to speak at them. It is harder to divine any kind of reply. And yet that is what I tried that January, so soon after my diagnosis. I did not always speak to the living at this time. I did not talk to Ben much about the common ground between us, in part because it did not feel like common ground any more. Our illnesses, his mortal but curable, mine incurable but a little more wayward in its progression, did not seem to be the same shape at all.

The person I wanted to talk to was Gene, however, and the problem was simple: Gene had died. Somehow, he had been dead for ten years. He was a dear friend, so he still lived on somewhat in the world around me, a tap on the shoulder when I saw something that reminded me of him or that I knew we had spoken about. But those taps had grown less frequent over time, and I would address him in my head less and less. There was less to tell him about.

Suddenly, though, I knew that I needed him. Selfishly, I felt that he had experience that I could learn from. He had made it deep into the territory where I now found myself. Before he had died, he had also been an incurable.

And so: 'Should I maybe take a trip?' I asked. 'With Leon.

See a bit of the world together?' Suddenly nervous: 'You know. Just the two of us?'

I was bathing Leon, a dark January evening with Sarah leaning in the doorway trying to put work out of her head. She had a glass of water in her hand, which she had brought me to take my pill with. Now that I had, and now that swift flames were racing across my shoulders and over my scalp, she was absent-mindedly sipping from the water herself, swilling it around her mouth like a wine-taster.

'Where would you go?' she asked. I almost replied, 'Boston, the English one.' Instead, I said, 'I was thinking about seeing Gene.' A pause. I realized that what I had said was not quite correct.

'Gene?' Sarah reached for the name. 'Isn't he dead?'

'I certainly hope so, darling,' I replied, teasing Leon's wet hair into short blonde spikes. 'We cremated him.'

Leon slapped my hand away and flattened her hair. Sarah gave me the weary look she had started to give me over the last few weeks. It was the look that said that she, at least, had noticed that I was approaching euphoria, and maybe it would be nice for us both to notice this together.

I explained that I had meant to say that I was thinking of seeing Brian, a friend of both Gene and mine from my first spell at university, spent further along the south coast. Another seaside town: Bournemouth. Brian had stayed put after the rest of us had left, and, earnest, generous, funny and sad, he was someone I didn't get to see enough.

'It would be good for us!' I said. 'Well, it would be good for me. I could take a day off work. Nobody will miss me. I haven't taken Leon anywhere by myself yet – not out and about.'

Sarah sat down on the edge of the toilet and watched me taking Leon out of the bath, wrapping her slippery fish body in a towel and fuzzing her hair, creating reluctant giggles. 'Why not?' she said at last, looking down at the glass in her hand. And then: 'Did you take your pill?'

'I think so,' I replied, but already I had no idea.

Still, why not indeed? That head rush of diagnosis was still expanding within me. It had lasted for a good few months or so, obliterating Christmas and rolling into January, making me feel like I was flying, arms outstretched, borne aloft by sheer energy and the belief I could outpace this unknowable catastrophe that I was suddenly expected to live with. I was put in mind of that line of Fitzgerald's – a note to himself in the unfinished manuscript of *The Last Tycoon*, and my favourite fragment of anything he wrote: 'My blue dream of being in a basket like a kite held by a rope against the wind.' The annotation for this reads 'Airplane Trip', and maybe I felt a little of that skymindedness, a little of the giddy, improbable early days of aviation.

Why not indeed? I was on new pills that shook me roughly every morning and evening, rubbing fire into the skin around my neck and my cheeks, like a good sharp headwind. And it seemed that MS might be more or less contained by this medication, angry lymphocytes lifted out of reach, to the upper atmosphere. The pills left me high, or rather MS left me high. High on the sheer impact of sudden change.

Really, what was I now? Was I afflicted? A few twinges and pangs aside, I didn't feel it yet. I felt like a survivor, a pioneer. An explorer. Here was a new world, a life altered, and I felt dangerously positive about my prospects. After years of caution, I was suddenly speaking too fast, too loud, at every opportunity, and people let me because I had told them all, in great detail, what was happening to me. I was the bright light of every conversation – at least I was in my own recollection afterwards. Which generally doesn't bode well.

I was kidding myself that I had already started to understand my illness. At night, tingling in the darkness, I felt like I was hovering high above the earth, interesting possibilities stretching in every direction. And now a new guide had appeared.

'Remind me who Gene was?' asked Sarah, the night before I left to see Brian.

'Gene was a friend from university,' I said. 'A mature student, nearly twenty years older than me and the rest of us. He died about a decade ago. He was a renal patient.'

Yes. Gene was a guide. He had seen the place I was heading into, and maybe, if I could get a bit closer to him, or closer to the memory of him, he might have something important to tell me about it.

I was in the kitchen with Sarah, loading a bag with snacks for the trip: chopped fruit in little boxes, rice cakes, bread sticks. Another bag contained nappies and nappy bags. ('Do you think I should take anything for Leon as well?' I had asked, looking at the nappies, as I always asked. It struck me that my diagnosis probably made this joke less amusing.) There would be a pushchair, several changes of clothes. Leon was no longer being breastfed during the day, but she would have long snoozes and there would be disasters. This last point was freshly minted in my mind. The day before the trip, Leon had fallen in a puddle of dog pee by the library. Somehow, I had changed her while chatting to Janey in a nearby Starbucks, swapping over trousers, disinfecting skin, and managing to order a mocha at the same time. Euphoria has its benefits.

'Are you sure you want to do this?' Sarah asked.

'It's only one day,' I said. 'And I've had her at weekends loads when you've been at work.' Besides, I could have added, I want to test myself with Leon. Seventeen months old all of a sudden and I'm not sure I'd really taken on any parental challenges. Not any of the kind that tested my concept of myself as a decent parent.

★

In the dark of our tiny porch, she catches a flash of colour as I fling my orange scarf around my shoulders. I shrug on too many bags and back out of the door, bumping the pushchair from ragged carpet to uneven paving. ('Crazy paving?' I had once asked Sarah. 'Demented,' she had replied, and we agreed to put it on the long list of things to fix.) Seconds before, just as we left the warmth of the living room, MS reached forward in silence and placed a shushing finger against the base of my neck. I can still feel it there, pressing below the thyroid as we head to the bus stop. I will feel it all day, a narrowing of the throat that may be gone tomorrow or in a week's time as the whimsy of this thing dictates.

As we wait at the stop I fuss with Leon's coat, drawing it close against the wind that rushes in, stinging, carrying the chill of the sea. She is awake, frowning with cold, and she shrugs and squirms away from me as I move her hair around and try to clip it — not that there is much to clip yet. On the bus, she brightens, and by the time we are going through the barriers at the station and bumping up into a carriage, I'm feeling pretty positive about our chances. Our first trip together: I should take a picture on my phone, but it feels like it might force an end to this moment we are in, pushchair stowed and bags wedging us tight by the window.

She's happy. She is sitting on my lap, hands flat on the table, taking in the new sights. I find my pill in among pocket change. 'Mennen,' she notes brightly. Pride and grief that she knows that word: *medicine*. Minutes later I feel the prickly heat just below the surface of my skin. It is still working. It is still doing something.

Leon babbles at me, except that this is old thinking, and the noises she makes are no longer meaningless babble, and maybe haven't been for some time. 'Whaddat?' she demands, pointing out of the window. 'Telegraph poles,' is the answer. 'Fields.' 'A power substation?' She has a daunting supply of 'whaddats' stored up, and my responses are already becoming speculative. Children show you a new world, Dad had warned me. It turns out they also show you the gaps you never filled in the old one.

She has changed so much, even in the few months since she first staggered across the living room towards me. Her light dandelion fuzz of hair has become something approaching a style – blonde and short, a *Rosemary's Baby* cut. Her newborn moon-face has started to take its own shape: she has cheekbones now and a gently rounded chin. Her huge eyes now narrow with laughter because something is actually funny, or squint, frowning, at new sights. She walks everywhere she can; she eats everything she can.

And there is so much more to her world: she is inquisitive, searching, quick to anger and quick to forget. There is something monumental at work, and as she stands on my knees, leaning into the window, held aloft by my hands in hers, like I'm her puppeteer, I realize what it is. She laughs at a field of frosty scrub and turns to see if I'm laughing too – at the way the sunlight settles in the icy mud like glitter. Suddenly, I understand this: she's no longer a baby, a creature to nurse, a thing to take around and keep out of trouble. She's a companion. The two of us are going somewhere together, and I am no longer Daddy Chloroform, tasked only with sleep.

And when she does sleep there is a chance to reflect on where I am going, and why. The frosty morning has endured, coating the world moving past the window with a thin white fur: a little Manhattan of teetering wooden pallets on the outskirts of the docks, those gloomy mounds of speckled earth on a winter farm, empty fields giving way to silent rows of solar panelling. This is, it occurs to me, a journey into the past, headed between two towns that are linked for me because I went to university in each of them. I remember moving to Brighton and post-grad life in 2000 and feeling not that things were finally starting, but that I was somehow suspended again, in a holding pattern between more substantial moments. University had felt real the first time around; the second time it felt like a rerun, an indulgence too far. And I feel a little suspended again now, after the verdict of diagnosis but awaiting the verdict on the drugs I'm taking every day – drugs that might be changing a trajectory that I am possibly just starting to understand.

Looking back at my first university, it is very clear that there were three years of Gene that I wasted. We were at university together, but we weren't really there together. I doubt we noticed each other much in large classes, filled with chatter and scribbling. Still, we were all drawn there for the same thing at least: a degree, improbably, in the art of scriptwriting. A degree in fantasy.

Gene was older than me, but so was practically everyone back then. I am a summer baby, and so I was still used, in my early twenties, to being the youngest person in every situation I found myself in. Gene was a mature student, inching towards forty. Even Brian was a year or two older than I was. Brian was on the same course as Gene and me, but again, I didn't really meet him until it was all over.

I loved university: we worked like crazy, writing both for coursework and to learn the art of observation, jotting down everything that happened to us in little notebooks we had been instructed to carry in a back pocket or a bag. I remember watching the coursework pile up, and I remember stacking notebooks on my desk, ten, fifteen, twenty of them filled with things I had spotted, things that had occurred to me as I wandered about. It felt like all of this work was building to something, and then the course finished, we all graduated, and it turned out that there had been no real conclusion. Act three, as I would have put it at the time, had lacked a climax, and had

also been lumbered with an obscure and circuitous denoue-
ment. The protagonists had not learned much. Action had not
become character. It was hard to know how to interpret things,
other than to realize that I was suddenly an adult, allegedly,
adrift in a world of adult things and trained for precisely
nothing.

So of course I plotted a return to university, to the one thing
I now knew how to do. But before that there was a year to fill:
with a job in an insurance office in which I was now, rather
worryingly, no longer the youngest person there; and with the
only friendly faces I saw around town – Gene and Brian. Three
students who had all stayed put when everyone else had gone.
We fell together naturally.

Brian, I discovered, was generous and kind and gloriously
maudlin. In his early twenties he already suspected that life had
passed him by, that the best was behind him, and so he was
looking for people to spend the afterlife with. He had a job at
the cinema and got the three of us into free screenings. We
worked as a trio. The age gap wasn't weird. It just meant that
Gene knew a lot more about movies and books and life than
Brian and I did. He was willing to put up with us, anyway.
Brian was tall and dark-haired and rather beautiful; Gene was
more like me, rumpled and slightly bowed. His soft voice
meant you had to lean in to hear him speak. Did we realize he
was dying? I can't remember. Maybe Brian would.

The ideal place for coffee is part of a railway station. I have always
felt this. There's something about the stillness amid the bustle,
something about standing and stopping as a great crowd flows
around you. One of my best railway coffee stops was Ramses
Station in Cairo on an undergrad trip twenty years ago: citi-
zens of the world drinking beakers of sweet black tea and eating
brittle, quietly disappointing cakes on their way to places I

would never visit myself, a sun-stained ruffle of Baedeker pages to everything I saw and touched and smelled.

Another favourite is less dramatic, a place on the south coast of England, part of a station you would never choose to stop at. It's a narrow, echoing space with fraying carpets and clanking china. The walls are carved red brick rising and rising into shadow as they become lost in the gloom of the ceiling. I have been coming here once or twice a year since the days when people could smoke indoors, and when I look up to those ceilings I still seem to see them through a grainy fog of twisting ash.

An ideal place for a coffee, and a promising place to raise the dead.

I have never brought Leon here, but after a speculative grump on alighting from the train, this strange establishment calms her. I find a highchair, an improbable discovery in a place as resolutely Victorian as this, and she sits, pulping banana between her fingers and staring about with bright, happy eyes.

And then Brian joins us, tall and romantic, with shiny black hair and grey eyes permanently narrowed at the world, lips made for exhaling weary disappointment. I am shocked, as ever, by his handsomeness and how gentle he is in his movements. He is used to children – I think his mother works at a nursery – and Leon instantly reflects his ease, watching as he wiggles his fingers back and forth and covers his eyes, then his mouth, cycling through bizarre expressions until she has forgotten her pulped banana and sees her life's work – or at least that of the next few hours – as watching everything this strange man does.

'I remember the white-suit story the most,' says Brian once we have sat down and talked about how long it has been – and how much longer it has been since Gene died. I want to ask about Gene's illness, but I suspect you cannot approach that directly, so we're talking about this instead. 'He loved *12 Angry Men*, that film where Henry Fonda is very righteous and wears this white linen suit. His mum asked what he wanted for Christmas one year, and he really wanted a white suit like Henry Fonda's. He tried to explain it to her, but then he had to back away from it.'

'The suit?' I ask.

Brian nods. 'Basically, he thought his mum was going to get him a *Saturday Night Fever* suit by accident.'

Conversation stutters. I have not seen Brian in a long time, and we have forgotten how to sync our rhythms of speech together. I hunt, slight panic building, for a way to keep us talking, or I fear he might just get up and walk away. I have no idea why I fear this. While I hunt, the spectre of Gene wearing a disco leisure suit hovers between us and will not be banished.

Were we an unusual trio, I ask, Brian and Gene and I? Gene was from a different generation. 'And he was a different speed,' remembers Brian. 'He could walk, but he was quite slow and shuffling. He had to sit down every few minutes. Eventually, you'd just match his pace.' He thinks about this. 'It was great, actually. You'd notice much more of the world that way.'

Yes. I am starting to remember some of this stuff now. Inching down the street with Gene. You had so much more time to talk to him, because it took so long to get anywhere. He never complained about it. But also, he was never apologetic – a trait I had not noticed at the time, but which I now realize I admire.

'He used to say it was his job, being ill,' Brian says. 'He said the only problem was it didn't pay very well.' He trails off, and I look up from wiping Leon's hands just quickly enough to see an awkward look cross those grey eyes, a sense that he thinks he might have touched on unexplored territory between us. New territory. I have not seen Brian since my diagnosis – I *texted* him the news, which was classy – and now I understand that while my conception of myself is in flux, his conception of me, of our relationship, is probably in flux too.

'Do you remember the leather jacket he wore?' asks Brian suddenly. Yes! I have a memory of old brown leather, cracked to gold around the collar, of pockets that sagged like the lining was torn. 'Do you remember the shirt with the dragon on it?' No, not at all.

'Here is the problem,' I say to Brian. 'I have such a warm sense of this man, and in my current state I have this idiotic feeling that he might have something to say to me, something to guide me through whatever's going on with me. But I don't know what my memories actually add up to. I can't seem to *see* him any more, as he was. And the one picture I have of him – he's holding a baby, his niece – I have put on a high shelf because he's holding the baby so badly Sarah keeps laughing at it.'

'You feel like you're forgetting?' asks Brian, wincing slightly. 'Is that MS?'

This is the only time that he mentions MS in our conversation. He may be older than me but he's committed to youth: dancing, DJing, job in a supermarket. His latest thing is running marathons.

'I honestly don't think so,' I say. 'I think it's just – what – ten years, almost to the day, since he died. I'm forgetting everything from ten years ago. It's all just fading.'

'I can remember some helpful things,' says Brian. 'Let's walk?' He nods at Leon. 'She's almost done with her banana anyway.'

Amazingly, Brian wants to carry her. More amazingly, she is up for this, and so I push the pushchair through the cold streets while she sits merrily in his arms, visibly thrilled to be up high and a part of everything that's happening. And what's happening is Brian rebuilding Gene for us both, or trying to,

out of anecdotes, out of tiny pieces of memory. Right now, he
is explaining the classic elements of a Gene story: you must
have an objective, and a social fear, and the social fear must
scupper the objective.

'That's why he never got the white suit,' Brian explains. 'It's
a pincer movement, like Stalingrad. There's the fear that his
mum will get the wrong suit, and then the fear that he'll have
to wear the wrong suit regardless so as not to disappoint
his mum.'

Not disappoint, I think. Upset. Gene never felt like he had to
be anything to anyone else, but he was terrified of causing pain.

Brian searches for another story to confirm his narratology,
and so we get lost sifting through details. He loved cricket,
Gene – loved Shane Warne, the bowler. He loved gambling:
the first time I saw him after university he was coming out of a
bookie's with eight hundred quid he'd just won on an accumu-
lator. He always had a flutter going on something or other. He
was endlessly recalculating the date at which he would break
even. Last I heard it was going to be 2021.

He was political – political in a way that we weren't, old
enough to have been directly engaged with poll-tax riots and
Thatcher the Milk Snatcher. Even so, he was gentle, and
people were gentle around him. He sagged into chairs and then
sat forward when people spoke to him. He was quiet and alert.

I try to prod us back towards the thing I am suddenly far too
interested in. Gene's illness, did it weigh on him? Did he ever
talk about it with us? I mention a rare trip to Gene's house to
watch a film, in which we briefly ducked into the kitchen for
tea and I saw a landslide of blister packs on a sideboard. So
many pills, different sizes and colours, spilling over the coun-
ter. And Gene just brushing past them, saying: 'Do you still
take two sugars?'

Brian steers me out of the kitchen. He can't remember

anything about pills. Instead, he goes into the stuff I didn't know about, coming from the days after I left town for Brighton. He tells me about the time they used to spend playing pitch and putt together, about an unlikely Clint Eastwood impression. The time Gene bought Brian a T-shirt – *I Fought the Law and I Won* – after a tribunal at the cinema. This Gene sounds like a riot, but is it my Gene? I remember someone watchful and sometimes silent, perhaps separated from the rest of us by perspective. A grown-up around us children.

Maybe Brian remembers this Gene too. 'Do you remember the thing about the Age of Reason?' Brian asks, buckling Leon up and gesturing that he'd like to push her for a bit.

'The Age of Reason?' I ask.

'You'd been reading some Thomas Pynchon book set in the Age of Reason,' Brian says. 'And you were mad keen on it, and going on about how you belonged there, and maybe all of us did. I was talking about how I fancied the wigs and the coats and all that, and then Gene just laughed.

'And he said, "I'd be dead in the Age of Reason."'

'Christ.'

'It was one of the only times he really talked about what was happening, about the transplants he'd had that hadn't worked, about the dialysis every other evening. He laughed. He wasn't upset, but it was one of those moments when you saw where he was.'

'Are you writing much these days?' I asked.

Before I headed off, we found a coffee shop with toy blocks, and pretty quickly we abandoned our drinks and were just playing with Leon on the carpet. Brian was deeply involved in peekaboo, a game that Leon intermittently understood, and loved even when she lost its rhythms, laughing theatrically each time Brian's face appeared from behind his hands, slapping

her palms against the ground and giggling until I thought she
might be sick.

'Nothing,' Brian said.

A wound. Brian had been the busiest writer I knew back at
university – and this was supremely impressive since he worked,
for the first two years, on a computer-typewriter combo that
stored only thirty pages of work in memory, meaning that on
long projects he relentlessly had to retype old sections when he
wanted to rework them and reprint them.

Even after we left university, Brian was endlessly hacking out
pages. He wrote a Mills & Boon book to a formula, but abandoned the formula halfway through when he read *Catch-22* for
the first time and found himself transforming a tale of love in a
supermarket – the title was 'A Walk Down the Aisle' – into a
dark screwball examination of life's inherent absurdities. Next
up, he wrote a series of detective novels based on a beloved lec-
turer of ours, who had always seemed needlessly hard-boiled.
They were the kinds of books where baddies were forever chuck-
ing the hero through plate-glass windows. I remember Brian
coming up to me at the cinema one day, face glowing. A literary
success: he had just conceived of a scene in which the baddies
closed an open window and then chucked the hero through it.

It felt like we could have talked here, about how our lives
had changed. But why talk about it? There was coffee, and a
baby rolling around and playing peekaboo like it was the new-
est, most exciting thing in the world. Which it was. And was
she even a baby any more? I would have to ask Sarah.

Instead, after I'd changed Leon, I prepared everything for
the journey back. I felt a slight sense of failure. I had convened
a sort of seance, and yet Gene had failed to turn up. We had
traded stories and the table had maybe rattled a few times, but
the spare chair we had placed next to us remained empty.

We walked out into the cold. I got ready to shoulder Leon's

buggy up the hill, and I saw Brian frozen, locked in a sudden memory in front of his car. 'Gene had that thing, that little cardboard disc that allowed him to park anywhere because he was a disabled person,' he said. 'Do you remember? Do you remember the way he used to set the dial on it and then frisbee it on to the dash?'

He laughed. 'Always a little flourish with him. Always a little mockery to it.'

Leon slept on the way back, and as she drifted off, Gene returned to me, slowly, tentatively. I willed him to me with effort. Forget the stories, I told myself. Forget the things I know he liked and the things I know he often did. Clear your mind of that and search for what you actually remember.

And then there he was. Not the Gene of anecdote we had been pondering all afternoon – this was Gene as he was across the table from you, body sagging but mind wonderfully sharp and playful.

What I remember of people is their hands. I hate to meet people's eyes, so I watch the rest of them, and the hands are the true stars of the body, beautiful and expressive. Gene's hands were particularly memorable, elegant movements, skin yellowed by disease and nicotine, fingernails wide and flat and thick, popping pills out of blister packs, scratching the back of his neck as he thought about something difficult and abstract, or crafting filterless cigarettes with the aid of a little box – both storage tin and rudimentary roll-up factory – that I remember being fascinated with.

'Like it?' he said to me once, opening the box and showing me the mechanism.

'I don't get it,' I said. Inside, the box was just a flap of loose canvas and a thick metal pin. And yet when he put in paper, one edge wetted, and added tobacco, and then fired the mechanism by closing the lid, the whole thing came together and he got a cigarette out of it.

He lit up and puffed clean white smoke. In his last years, he decided to be dapper, so he wore a shirt and tie everywhere, rumpled, of course, as if he were a private eye who had to sleep on his office sofa. This would have been towards the end, I think. Maybe a year or two left. He may have been thirty-eight.

'My nurse likes this tin,' he said. 'The two of you always want to see it. She can never get how it works either.'

'Are you allowed to smoke in hospital?' I asked. 'Aren't there oxygen tanks around and that sort of stuff?'

'I can't smoke in there, but I guess I just like rolling them,' he said. He would have reached for his tea now – a half cup. He could only have half cups, and I got very good at making them, getting the milk just right. He loved tea. Loved a Coke. He loved a drink, and – yes! – he used to get very angry when he watched movies and people were offered drinks and turned them down. Renal failure meant he was always thirsty.

I had forgotten the tea, the amused anger at the films. For weeks after he died, I kept making half cups of tea out of instinct. And I had forgotten the nurse. I don't think he became dapper for her. I think he became dapper because here was a little, throwaway thing he could control. But I can imagine him smoothing his shirt for her, leaving his tie loosely knotted and carefully, artfully, raked to one side, as if by accident.

In his house: New York on the wall in black-and-white photographs. Those pills in the kitchen. Yellow hands marked with deep purple stains. Gentle hands reaching for those pills.

'Gene!' I said aloud in the train carriage, so loudly that I woke up Leon. Had I been asleep myself? 'Hope not,' I said, out loud again, thinking of parenting. Leon yawned at me and smiled.

Getting home felt like an achievement: a whole day trip with my daughter, and both of us making it back. But I also sensed something in Brian's easy way with Leon, his instant camaraderie with her, which shamed me slightly. 'I should have taken her out before now,' I said to Sarah as I eased Leon back into the bath that night. It seemed to be all bathing in Leon's first few years: Leon and I, the two of us peering at each other as her toys bobbed around her in the bubbles, me kneeling by the tub the way my mum had once knelt by the tub.

'You've had her by yourself, and that's not bad,' said Sarah.

'Yeah, but you've taken her all over the place, and I've just discovered it's not actually that hard. I feel like I'm coming to everything too late. Like I'm a Victorian parent who's all lofty and weird about everything.'

Leon burped at me, and a bubble came out of her mouth. 'Fruit?' she asked speculatively, thinking of dinner.

'Not in the bath, darling,' I countered. See? A Victorian.

Later, Leon in bed, Sarah asked me as I eased on to the sofa, 'Did you get any closer to him?'

'Gene?' I clarified. 'A lot of memories. Him being funny, him being ill. I thought that would all be bound up together more. We only knew him when he was ill, but maybe we weren't really paying attention as much as we should have.'

'What was he like before he was ill?' Sarah asked.

I opened my mouth and then shut it. I realized I had never really thought about this before.

'I think he was a bit of a hero,' I finally said, frowning. 'We went to his funeral, Brian and I. We met all these people who had known him his whole life, and they all wanted to know what we made of him. We were so much younger than everyone else there, so they were curious about him as we knew him – curious about his later years.'

I thought back to Golders Green, a rainy day that ended with us lost in a park somewhere, looking for a bench that had been commemorated for Gene. It was the sort of strange adventure Gene himself would have driven us to. I think we probably got the bus.

'I saw a picture of him when I was at the funeral,' I said. 'An early picture – his twenties, probably. I didn't recognize him. He got arthritis and then he got renal failure, one-two, falling like that. But before that, he was this rangy guy who loved cricket, who was the star bowler of his team. They told me, just before he got ill, he had this one year at cricket where he couldn't fail. Everything he did just worked. He smashed it. He was funny and vivid, and you saw it all in that face, uncreased, unblemished. He was a rabble-rouser. He liked anarchy.

'He seemed worldly,' I said. 'And that wasn't because he'd travelled. It was because he'd been sick. He told me this story of when he got really bad blood poisoning because of his kidneys, and he got confused. He didn't know what was going on, and his doctor sat down and drew these circles, and said, "Gene, these are clock faces. Write in the numbers."

'He wrote one, two, three, and stopped. His doctor said, "Any more?" So he wrote four, five, six, and stopped again. And so on and so on. All around the clock.'

I told Sarah then. I told her that I felt Gene had something to say to me, but I couldn't hear it.

'Like a secret?' she asked, eyes laughing.

'He told me a few secrets,' I said. 'He told me about the nurse. He told me – he leaned forward once and whispered, "I never need to cut my hair. It just doesn't grow so I leave it and always say yes when people ask if I've had it cut." And he told me about his secret plan for if he got better.'

'What was that?' Sarah asked.

'He was going to go to New York,' I said. 'Do the whole writer thing. It would have suited him. He finished things, but he would go back and tinker. He was almost always 70 per cent through a project. He said that was what being a writer was all about – the first act done, the second act done, third act tentatively in there, but having a break to think about tying it all up.'

'How did he die?' Sarah asked, after a while.

And I had to think about it.

I have always known how Gene died: renal failure. But I'd forgotten the particulars. And suddenly they came back, and it was Christmas again, a cold white day in late December, and I was splayed on a sofa at a friend's house in Camberwell. We were watching one of those cable TV history programmes with terrible re-enactments filmed on an impossible budget. This was the football game between the Germans and the Brits on Christmas Day in the trenches. Actors playing Germans were wobbling up out of their trench bearing a Christmas lantern that looked like it was made of old coat hangers. Our boys were lowering their prop guns and trying to work out whether this was a devious ploy or not.

The phone rang. I was holding the phone and listening. A voice on the other end I didn't recognize: a cockney nan, scratchy and garbled, and when the line cleared she was saying, 'It's Gene's mum.'

I knew then. I had been waiting for this call. Gene had gone into hospital. He'd been given a final chance at a kidney transplant. It had come together at the last moment and it was ludicrously risky. If it worked, he'd have his old life back. If it didn't, he'd be as good as dead.

It hadn't worked, by the sounds of it, but Gene was still alive. He was in hospital and somehow he was doing okay.

'I think the hospital he was in was miles away from his home – he was in Bristol, which was the hospital that had offered him the transplant. I talked to him once over those hospital phones, but he wasn't able to focus. I tried to ring again

the next day and the next day, but the phone wasn't working
any more – it just went to busy.'

(Admission: I was glad I couldn't get through, as the person
on the phone didn't sound like Gene. Now I would kill for that
call, on the most crackling line, with the most distracted version of Gene at the other end. 'What would you say?' Sarah
asked when I eventually told her this. 'Nothing much,' I said.
'There was nothing unsaid between us. I'd ask him about his
recent winnings.')

Then Brian called on Boxing Day morning. Gene had died on
Christmas Day. Mum started to cry and I was furious with her.
For a few days I was furious at everything. I sat playing my old
Game Boy Micro in the freezing garage room at Mum's house,
fuming as I lay on a tiny bed that my feet stuck out the end of.

As I told the story I felt it all again. Memories that I had not
returned to, and so they were fresh, like Ben having a seizure in
his bedroom. Gene died all over again. He died every time I
thought of that fucking tin of his, with the clever mechanism
inside that somehow managed to roll cigarettes. And still I
couldn't see what I was looking for. Suddenly, awash in sheer
frustration, I wanted to cry.

'You looked up to him,' said Sarah. 'And he knew what it
meant to be an incurable.'

I nodded and leaned into her. My head was on her shoulder,
her voice coming to me from above. She started to stroke
my hair.

'But he can't do this for you. He can't take you through this.'
She forced me to look at her. 'And he shouldn't.'

'He shouldn't,' I mumbled. I agreed.

'If he were here, what would he say to you?' Sarah asked me.
I thought for a while.

'He would say: "Remember I was more than this,"' I said.
And more, I thought: he would tell me that illness is not

always the end of life, and even when it is, it is not always the point of it.

Is that why he went for that last transplant? I never really understood the last transplant, not that it was any of my business, and I still didn't understand it now. What I did understand was that over the last few weeks I had promoted Gene's illness to the forefront of his identity, and it didn't really belong there. For the last few weeks I had tried to raise Gene's ghost to talk to him about death. That's what it was, wasn't it? I didn't want to ask him about life as an incurable so much as I wanted to ask him about life in the vivid presence of death. But all of my memories of him – jokes, cricket, even that white suit he never asked for – all of my memories of him lead back to life.

'He's a memory,' said Sarah. 'He doesn't have to be a resource.'

'There was a weightiness to him,' I said, and in my mind I was now watching the rest of that stupid re-enactment show. The Germans and the Brits playing a tentative game of football in the mud, the tempo increasing with each kick, the awareness – even on this tacky programme – that this good thing that was coming together could not last. 'Not to him,' I said. 'To our dealings with him. An awareness that he had a far more profound sense of perspective that we found a bit awesome.' I notice now that people sometimes assume I have a wider perspective. Erroneously in my case, because my concerns have remained enduringly trivial.

'He was forty,' I said.

'He never had kids,' I added, although Sarah hadn't asked, and wouldn't have.

Death feels so ridiculous. Every time someone I know dies, that's what comes back to me in the shock: how ridiculous it is that we are meant to believe that someone so vividly *close* is suddenly out of reach for good.

Still, the dead live on, I have discovered, occupying the corner of my vision, the very edge of the window, the first movement of a double-take.

When I take off my glasses in a crowd, the people around me start to change. My brain starts to fill in the blanks and turn these strangers into people I know. In the years immediately after Gene died, I used to perform this trick now and then in order to see him again, which is why I know that there's no better place to try it than at the long corridor through the middle of St Pancras.

St Pancras is the best, because the corridor is long and white with a great vanishing point. Shortly after my trip to see Brian, I went there with Leon one afternoon and stood, rocking her back and forth in her pushchair, as we waited for a train to come in. Any train, just as long as it brought that great exhalation of passengers with it.

The trains came. I pushed Leon into the centre of the corridor with me, and then I took off my glasses. In the brain, the dead can live – and Gene did. He was all around me again, bowed, shuffling, looking up with a laughing smile, ready to tell me about the last film he had watched.

But it is an illusion. Gene can approach, but he can never get too close. The illusion breaks down and we're surrounded by strangers again. And so the dead continue to teach the living.

'I Only Observe, Nothing More'

Jean-Martin Charcot and the discovery of MS

You can see it today on Google Maps, slung along the left bank of the Seine. 'Pitié-Salpêtrière' reads the marker that hovers over this vision of order rendered in stone, cream-coloured wings stretching away from a central dome. Somebody has helpfully added a note: 'Teaching hospital with turbulent history'.

It was a gunpowder factory, then a dumping ground for the poor and the mad. A prison for prostitutes that was notable for the number of its rats. In the 1650s, the Salpêtrière became a hospital, steadily growing in size and surviving a raid during the Revolution. It was here in the 1860s that Jean-Martin Charcot, often working with his colleague Edmé Félix Alfred Vulpian, would turn the study and classification of neurological disease into a science.

I try to picture Charcot at work, during the morning consultations, sitting in a small office lit by a single window, the walls painted black. In this spare, slightly menacing environment, he would watch his patients as they stood before him. He rarely spoke; sometimes he might tap his hand on the table as his dark eyes took everything in. In his later years, as his fame grew, he would give lectures on the diseases he was uncovering, lectures that brought in doctors visiting from as far away as Japan and the US, as well as journalists, writers and theatrical stars. He taught Freud for a brief but pivotal period in the 1880s and remained a huge influence on the psychoanalyst. Before all that, in the space of a few decades, he described Parkinson's disease and motor neurone disease. And he started, in 1868, by describing multiple sclerosis, or, to use the name he gave it, *la sclérose en plaques*.

Charcot was born in Paris in 1825, the eldest son of an artisan and carriage-builder. Growing up around artists, he considered a career as a painter, but medicine offered more money, and more scope for social advancement.

Initially an undistinguished student, by the time Charcot applied for internships he was described as being 'above average in his knowledge, capacity and zeal'. Zeal may have been the crucial factor for Charcot in his early years. He was an incredibly hard worker, publishing regularly and keeping track of international developments at a time when medicine was often parochial.

In 1861, he found an ideal laboratory: the Salpêtrière. At the time Charcot and Vulpian arrived (Charcot having previously interned there in 1852 while gathering data for his thesis on arthritis) the place was more of a small village than a hospital, home to five thousand female patients, most of them elderly, many of them muddled together under the umbrella diagnosis of epilepsy. Charcot and Vulpian immediately undertook an inventory of the people in their care, using new technologies such as photography to keep records. The initial aim was to separate the population by symptoms. Only then could they search for the underlying causes.

Charcot called himself a *visuel*. 'He was not a reflective man,' Freud wrote in a warm and reverent obituary. 'Not a thinker: he had the nature of an artist.' Charcot said of himself: 'All I am is a photographer' and 'I only observe, nothing more.' He also said: 'if you say [a doctor] is . . . a man who knows how to see, this is perhaps the greatest compliment one can make.'

The bedrock of Charcot's work at the Salpêtrière was the anatomo-clinical method, which he adapted from an approach popularized by René-Théophile-Hyacinthe Laënnec, the French physician who invented the stethoscope. Laënnec had a two-step system: he conducted a case study of the patient while they lived, and then cut them open once they had died, in order to match the symptoms he had witnessed to the physical evidence.

Here were two different approaches to seeing, and Charcot added a third: cellular pathology. He and his staff would observe a patient, sometimes for years, often keeping detailed diaries of the patient's life and their symptoms that have an almost literary feel to them. Once the patient had died, Charcot would conduct an autopsy. The objective was grand: to disentangle distinct neurological illnesses from groups of symptoms, and then to match each symptom to a specific lesion in the brain or on the spinal cord. To do that required patience, insight and a kind of benign predation.

It could be glacial work. 'Years of patient waiting were often necessary before the presence of organic change could be proved in those chronic illnesses that are not directly fatal,' wrote Freud. 'Only in a hospital for incurables like the Salpêtrière was it possible to keep the patients under observation for such long periods of time.' It was not just the opportunity, though; it was the way it was done. '[Charcot] used to look again and again at the things he did not understand,' said Freud, 'to deepen his impression of them day by day, till suddenly an understanding of them dawned on him.'

Many doctors had spotted features of MS and offered partial descriptions of the disease, and some had even sketched the plaques that are formed in the central nervous system of an MS patient. What was missing was clarity and a systematic understanding that distinguished MS from other neurological illnesses. Charcot and Vulpian began by studying tremors, which meant that they needed to develop yet more ways of seeing. Sphygmographs, wrist-mounted devices that measured arterial blood flow, were adapted to record hand movements, and patients were asked to hold large plumes in order to make their shaking easier to interpret. With these tools, Charcot and Vulpian were able to separate MS from what was then called shaking palsy. (It would continue to be called that until Charcot eventually offered a fresh description and gave it the name Parkinson's disease, in honour of the eighteenth-century doctor who had published the best early work on the condition.)

What Charcot and Vulpian had noticed was that each disease had its own kind of tremor. Parkinson's patients exhibit a tremor while at rest. MS tremors, however, occur when the patient is trying to do something. These action tremors, or intention tremors, became part of Charcot's triad of symptoms to be used in the diagnosis of MS. (The other parts of the triad are nystagmus, which is a hectic involuntary movement of the eyes, and telegraphic speech, in which speech is reduced to simple noun-plus-verb sentences. Charcot soon realized, however, that in the muddle of possible symptoms MS trades in, his triad was not particularly authoritative.)

Once Charcot and Vulpian had distinguished the different types of tremor, they were able to see that action tremors were often accompanied by other symptoms. The two doctors noted the visual and sensory problems of MS, and even spotted the relapsing and remitting form of the disease. Steadily, they brought MS into the light.

Charcot remains a fascinating, contradictory character. I feel, in an indulgent way, as if I am one of his patients, so I long to understand him properly, to make the separate pieces of him fit together. His private writings show a man who is caring and intensely sensitive, and yet it has been claimed that he could be imperious with his patients, and that he paraded them at his lectures as if they were animals in his circus.

Still, few would question the brilliance of the diagnostic work he produced in his early study of neurological illness. Charcot had a hospital full of patients that he couldn't save. Nobody had been able to fully understand what was wrong with many of these people until he came along. In the case of MS patients, you could argue that nobody had been able to truly see them. Charcot may not have been able to save them, but he found a way to see them.

'We are sometimes reproached for conducting incessant studies on the major neurological diseases, which have, up to now, mostly been incurable,' Charcot once wrote. (There is often a splinter of defensiveness buried in his writing.)

> What use is it? It has almost come to the point where people have questioned whether this is really medicine . . . But can you picture this? 'Dear patient, I am a doctor, it is true, but unfortunately I can do nothing for you; you belong to the category of the rejected with which we do

not deal!' No gentleman, our responsibility is otherwise. Let us keep looking, in spite of everything. Let us keep searching. It is indeed the best method of finding, and perhaps, thanks to our efforts, the verdict we will give to such a patient tomorrow will not be the same that we must give this patient today.

6. The Ghost on the Green

Leon was having a baby.

I learned this on waking one day in February, Leon and Sarah already sitting up in bed, having had what amounted back then to a conversation. Sarah turned to me and told me what I had missed. Congratulations were due: the baby was going to be a girl. Leon looked at me and nodded, frowning, her face suggesting she understood the weight of responsibility involved in all of this.

The baby would be coming from her grandparents – Sarah's parents – who lived nearby and looked after her a couple of days each week now that Sarah had returned to work part-time. The baby would be made of brown plastic and cloth. The baby would be called Poppy. I can't remember the exact words Leon used to tell us about Poppy; her vocabulary was grow-ing, but she was still yet to put together true sentences. Even so, she made her point well enough. We were all expectant. And then one evening, when Sarah's mum was dropping Leon off at the house, the baby was suddenly there with her.

'Is this Poppy?' I asked. Leon nodded, but ducked any more questions about the birth by shushing us: Poppy was asleep. 'Do you want to lay her down somewhere?' asked Sarah. I stood in a doorway, smugly delighted with the obvious care with which Leon held her baby and rocked her. This, after all, was our own parenting reflected back at us. I was warmed by its glow.

'Leon,' I said, eager to draw the moment out, to extend the radiance of our parental brilliance a little longer. 'Shall we get Poppy to bed before we have dinner?'

Sadly, that word – *dinner* – was one of Leon's favourites. On hearing it, some ancient instinct took over and she immediately changed focus. In the single beat of a heart she flung Poppy across the room and raced to her highchair.

Sarah and I stared at Poppy, upside down following a head-on collision with the skirting board. We were both silent. We were both thinking about parental brilliance.

In the days that followed, however, Leon was a surprisingly gentle mother. Often, she was gentle to the point of parody. When taking Poppy to bed at night, she would cradle her in her arms and walk so slowly across the room that even the cats got bored of following her around and wandered off to attack the furniture instead. Granted, Poppy's bedtime was also Leon's bedtime, so she had an incentive to drag it out, but she would also leap up every morning, pull back the covers and find Poppy, upside down again, face impacted in the mattress – every co-sleeper's nightmare – and chatter about how much she had missed her while she slept. I would always stop whatever I was doing when I saw Leon embarking on a moment of comical, prolonged tenderness. Since bringing Leon back from our visit to Brian, I had sensed worry creeping into my relationship with her – a fretful sadness that I could not quite pin down.

But there was nothing sad about watching her with Poppy. It never ceased to be a delight.

I awoke one February morning on a strange planet. I stayed for a couple of weeks. During the days I would see one sun nudging another across the sky; when night came, I would go to sleep beneath interlocking moons.

Diplopia had arrived, more commonly known as double vision, and while I had been expecting it – it is one of MS's trademark moves, due to the heavy myelination along the optic nerves – it was still a shock to experience it.

Coming soon after my journeys with Leon to see Brian, and then Gene, diplopia shattered the world into two intermingling images. Things in the foreground remained sharp and singular, but my new eyes jumbled the horizon, making the church spire outside my office window a shifting thing that seemed, whenever I moved, to trail a ghost behind it, at times all but merging with its own translucent form and then pulling away.

Luckily my working life revolved around screens, so I could just lean in and get close to the game I was playing or the text I was fumbling to put together and my eyes would be powerless to disrupt things. I would stumble occasionally as I wandered around the office, and I found myself getting very tired in the afternoons, but each morning I experienced a rush of energy that allowed me to rattle out thousands of words, and only a few hundred of them would be typos. 'Can you still do this stuff?' an editor asked me, concerned, when he found me one day at around three taking a nap on the sofa in the mini video studio we have set up at the back of the office. In truth, I wanted to say, I can *only* do this stuff. I have the perfect job for MS: sedentary, lots of chairs to slump in and games to pick away at, no thought to consider bigger than one that can fit into a thousand words. If I had come down with this ten years earlier, when I was pretending to work in the IT department of a health insurance company, I don't know how I would have managed. I don't know how other people manage, and I know that I should.

The bus I got to work, meanwhile, a bus which usually had BRIGHTON MARINA written on the side, now clanked to a stop beckoning me to BRIDGE MAR MARNIMAR – a location that it was hard not to like the sound of. Sarah was very excited about the bus at this point. She was still obsessed with the sea near our house and the strange metal creatures that lived there.

Construction had finally begun on a wind farm just off the coast, and the huge alien shapes of rigs now appeared along the horizon as we rattled into town. These rigs put temporary legs down into the sea, so they seem to float above the waves in silhouette. 'I wish you could see them like I see them,' I said to Sarah one day. 'They're not just floating, they're drifting through one another.'

Beyond spooky boats and the prospect of a day in Bridge Mar Marnimar, diplopia prods a person towards considering the beauty of normal functional sight. How does it work? What happens when it ceases to work? I wondered, at first, if part of my visual cortex, the part that reliably put two two-dimensional images together to create a single three-dimensional view of the world, might have been affected by MS.

The visual cortex is a wonder. Of all the brain's tricks, this one, to me, feels the most improbable: intricacy undertaken at speed. When light hits the photosensitive cells of the retina, it is transformed into an electrochemical message that is sent, via the thalamus, to the visual cortex at the back of the brain to be processed. The visual cortex is divided into many different regions, each of which handles a different aspect of the image, perceiving colour, say, or motion, or fixing the position of the object in view. I can't help but imagine this working a bit like pinball, like a beautiful pinball table built of gleaming order. The ball bearing races through the inside of the machine, pinging from one bumper to the next, all of which apply their own kind of spin or backspin. Onwards, and then out.

The problem for me was largely mechanical. The likely culprits were not the visual-processing pathways leading to the occipital lobe, which houses the visual cortex, but rather the nerves that supply the muscles which operate the eyes like pulleys. My eyes were no longer perfectly aligned, and this meant that the images the visual cortex was trying to put together had ceased to overlap as cleanly as they usually did. My perceptions were becoming harder to mesh.

I was not prepared for how tiring this was. In defiance of my shattered view of the world, one weekend Sarah took me and Leon to IKEA, a place that we both love wholeheartedly and without question. IKEA, the church of new beginnings, where young couples make tentative plans as they wander the aisles with measuring tape.

IKEA, alas, turned out to be exactly the wrong proportions for somebody who has trouble with the horizon.

We survived the little mock bedrooms of the first few areas beautifully – these spaces have always been my favourite, even if the pragmatic Scandi utopianism they preach has not entirely survived its collision with the crumbling realities of my own house. But then IKEA opens up and grows expansive.

My new enemy had a name: the Strandmon. I had never seen such Strandmon. IKEA's glorious 1950s wingback armchair, a masterwork of tasteful retro design, blessed with fine lumbar support and capable of transforming even the least reflective of sitters into a Victorian consulting detective, all crossed legs and templed fingers, was suddenly appearing in the showroom as if through a circus mirror, tangling and blending with myriad copies of itself, distorting, fragmenting, re-emerging intact. Everywhere I looked, Strandmon danced past Strandmon, colours shifting, shapes colliding, wings touching wings, legs sliding through legs, an elegant chair suddenly eager to trip itself up.

I felt woozy, so I had to sit down, wresting a nearby Strandmon out of the shimmering, rippling mass of its duplicates long enough to perch on it for a few seconds and steady myself.

'Don't even think of buying another,' said Sarah. 'The cats have already savaged the purple one.'

'It's dark blue,' I said, and then I staggered on.

Beyond the valley of the Strandmon, something far worse was happening to the Kallax bookcases, whose frames now converged with a fearful geometry, a futurist vortex of sustainable wood pulp that threatened to swallow Leon as we pushed her around in the shopping trolley. At the point where IKEA starts to deconstruct itself, dropping its customers into echoing flat-pack canyons where objects are reduced to slabs of golden cardboard stamped with the sheer, garbled intrigue of their brilliant names, my eyes were exhausted and I had to move with my head down, vision fixed on the smooth concrete floor that, thankfully, refused to play any tricks of its own.

But no, it's not that my eyes were exhausted. It's more that there was an angry congestion building somewhere behind them, in the parts of the brain that had to deal with the chaos my eyes were suddenly delivering. So much trouble, and all this from a shift in one eye – a shift, most likely, of much less than a millimetre. A shift so tiny that my eyeballs, viewed in IKEA bathroom mirrors, seemed perfectly normal as they tracked up and down, from left to right.

'It does not take much to start the unravelling,' I said to Sarah as we queued for the tills. Sadly, I often say this sort of cosily apocalyptic stuff by the time we have cleared the cardboard trenches of IKEA's final areas, so the full meaning of my words, such as it was, was lost.

Still. On the way home, I could not shake off this glimpse of the abyss that had opened up, so gapingly, in a suburb of Croydon. As the train headed back towards Brighton, we moved past converging fields, dark with February rain, and Gatwick, freshly fitted with dual runways that pushed against each other as they cast identical planes towards slightly different points on the horizon. Diplopia is dramatic, but it is not alarming so much as it is disquieting. It works its worst tricks internally, and in doing so it prods you towards the realization that your world is mediated on a number of intimate and invisible levels. You cannot see your own brain. Equally, you cannot see the tricks it works on you, because these are benign tricks designed to allow you to see in the first place.

The eyes are not things that work with your brain, like your hands, say, or the villi in your intestine, responding to orders from parts conscious and autonomic. The eyes are an extension of the brain – they are the bit of the brain we all get to see. This may account for how alien they can seem, these strange visitors hanging out in your face, a rubbery dome protecting the bizarre fantasy scene of your iris, stained the colours that nothing else in your body seems to be stained, and ridged with dark craters.

And perception should not always be trusted, even when it is working perfectly. The resolution of each human eye is inferior to the capabilities of the cameras in most smartphones, and even then only the macula and the fovea, the tiny areas at the centre of your vision, see things in any real sharpness at all. On top of that, as the information captured by the retinas is transformed into signals that are then processed by all those different parts of the visual cortex, a surprising amount of creative licence is applied. Signage in the street starts to say improbable things as the visual cortex makes guesses, and when I take off my glasses, the dead walk towards me. The brain fills in the gaps.

Diplopia fades, and like every other early neurological disaster, it seems less disastrous when you're looking back at it. For a while, as winter lingered into spring, double vision left glittering traces in me in the form of a sharp burst of panic every morning, which saw me leaping from bed and rushing to the window, not to see if February had brought snow, but to see if the buildings on the horizon were still firmly placed in the ground and separate from one another.

And it reminded me that I was still sick, in a way that I'm

ashamed to admit I found a little comforting at the time. Illness had kicked my sense of self into a swirling nebula of dust. Some aspect of the new personality that was cohering from this dust was clearly rooted in illness. Illness, or some primitive, imperfect idea of illness, was becoming a part of who I was, and this meant that during clear periods where MS retreated to an aching in the legs and a twitching underneath the skin, I was sometimes left feeling fraudulent as well as grateful. Everyone was suddenly being so nice to me about everything, and yet I hadn't really changed. This is a grim indulgence, of course, and I own its distastefulness. The same disease is rapidly ransacking people's lives and leaving them with no free time left to ponder such airy questions as who they are and who they might be becoming.

Still, diplopia was an energizing jolt. It reminded me that my world would be surprising from now on. It made it strange and fit for exploration. It also made me horribly anxious about what might come next.

I have told myself throughout all this that I have been saved, again and again, by a deeply ingrained curiosity – about my brain, about the way its mediation of my experiences, both healthy and unhealthy, affects the world I inhabit.

And yet there are times, going back over this story, that I see stark signs of a deeper incuriosity. One driven, inevitably, by fear. I was curious as to how diplopia might affect the aesthetics of IKEA store design, but I did not ponder what its presence in my life, after a month or so of exposure to the latest medication, might mean for the course of my disease, or its underlying power versus the not-inconsiderable power of the drugs newly stacked up against it.

Diplopia did not shake my belief that the pills were working – or rather that they were working and were also unmatched by the darker impulses of my own immune system. Medicine becomes a matter of faith if you don't really understand how it operates, and this faith was reinforced each morning, about thirty minutes after I had taken my pill, with that crimson rush of prickling heat that would touch off inside me. I had hospital appointments around this time, and I chose not to tell anybody I met with about my fortnight in Bridge Mar Marnimar – a fact that everyone I have since related it to finds incredible. But was it incredible? After all, I told myself, a fortnight is a fairly short space of time. Diplopia was not actually painful, aside from a slight headache. It was also very early in the course of my new medication; maybe it had already been cued up in advance, in some manner of speaking.

And anyway, I had already made my choice regarding my medication. I had found it difficult, and I did not want to have to make another choice again so swiftly afterwards.

The realization that MS is not simply a physical thing took a long time to set in. Every illness has its own emotional characteristics, I suspect. MS, I decided in my first few weeks, is a reflective thing – at least in this form, and in this case, and in its very early stages. *As if I would have any idea.* Still, I noted that I often seemed to retreat into the centre of my skull and had to peer out at the world *through* MS, as it changed everything in a thousand intangible ways related to sensation and perception. At first, MS was like wearing an odd pair of spectacles.

So it took a long time to realize that I was dealing with something not just wearying, but also potentially dehumanizing. Diplopia was crucial in this revelation. It prompted me to think about the world I had started to inhabit. And when I finally started to look around that spring, I told myself that I suddenly noticed the creeping symptoms of what the books and the websites sometimes called *cognitive decline*, apparent in terms of memory, general awareness, and a diminished ability to navigate anything that was not enormously straightforward.

How early on did this process begin? This is hard to say. Several months after my hands started tingling, but long before I started to suspect something serious was taking place, I was sitting on the carpet in the bedroom, trying to put an IKEA bed together. As I arranged the heavy parts of the bed, as I shook the screws out of their little plastic bags and into the saucer of a teacup, as I flipped through the instructions and made sure my tools were nearby, I felt something new.

Or rather I felt a new absence of something that had previously always been there.

Furniture construction, when I am in charge, is often a risky proposition. When I'm wielding the screwdriver and the Allen key, putting together anything bigger than a footstool suddenly belongs to the world of detective novels. *What is going to happen?*

With a bracing suddenness, I realized that I had no idea what I was doing. No idea at all. For a few minutes I went back and forth between the various pieces of flat-pack around me – the big parts of the bed, heavy as limbs; the screws describing modest arcs in their saucer as they settled; the thin pages of the instruction booklet – until I finally admitted that I could not get these pieces to converge in any way. I had an idea in my head: a bed. But I had no idea how the instructions related to the pieces laid out around me, and how all of that, in turn, would lead to the idea of a bed becoming tangible.

A pressure began to build in my head, starting with clogged ears and moving upwards until pain and annoyance prodded at my scalp from the inside. This was the hot pain of embarrassment and confusion, of exam papers that do not ask the right questions, of planes that have not waited for you on the tarmac when you have overslept. The paper, the images of the bed being put together: how did these instructions work? Why wouldn't they speak to me any more? Which elements did I start with? What did I need to put in my hands to begin?

I sensed a negotiation that was beyond me, and so I sloped into the living room, trailing defeat. Sarah had Leon snoozing on her lap. 'I can't do it,' I said. 'Something's wrong. I don't know how to start.'

'You never know how to start,' offered Sarah. 'Nobody does. Sit down and it will all come back to you.'

Sit down and it will all come back to you. I now sense nursing in that sentence — a little too much of it. And worse: this was not nursing emerging because I was ill. This was the nursing Sarah had had to adopt to get me from one end of a normal week to another when I was perfectly well. *Most of the things you should worry about come down to water,* I had said. What of the other things, though? Might they be the important things after all?

I got the bed made on my second attempt — the confusion had lifted and I suddenly knew exactly what to do. But now, months into a diagnosis, it seemed that the scuppering of the initial attempt to make the bed was not just my traditional reaction to flat-pack furniture — it was not anyone's traditional reaction to flat-pack furniture. Even Leon could have made a better go of it than I had. No, there had been a new shallowness there this time, a new inability to focus. It almost felt like there was less of me in my mind. Could that be MS?

In the weeks after diplopia faded, I grew increasingly clumsy. Not only was I still failing to connect with light switches, still failing to get keys into doors. That was beginner's stuff.

Suddenly I had two hands, and that felt like one too many. When carrying things, I would drop them unexpectedly and without reason, or I would knock one hand against the other and spill everything over myself. It is an odd feeling to knock one hand against the other. It's odd because it is rare, because it almost never happens. Your hands are given a degree of latitude to look after themselves. They have earned it, and until now my hands had always lived up to the challenge of their relative freedom.

Elsewhere, it seemed that my ability to deal with subtext was diminished. In the evenings, or if I was particularly tired, I found that I could no longer peer beneath the surface of what people were saying as easily as I had before. I was stuck in the literal.

Confused as I was, I knew that this was probably fascinating. TV drama was freshly dense with additional value: everything that happened was a wonderful shock; I failed to see even the most clumsy of telegraphed twists. Also, I failed to understand them even after they had occurred. 'What just happened?' I asked Sarah, halfway through *Revenge* one evening. *Revenge* is not a complex work. And yet here I was: I was asking back-from-the-kitchen questions, but I had not been out to the kitchen.

Is this a big thing or a little thing? This is one of the central questions as a case like mine develops. A case in which future horrors hang suspended and I am treated with great delicacy by the people around me, and yet I feel, at certain times, duplicitously healthy, disease contracted down to a slowness with words, or perhaps a few tiny dots of light that sting the very ends of my fingers.

But the big-thing-or-little-thing question is also something that exists inside the disease and occasionally emerges in strange ways. I will be sorting through the friendly jumble of laundry, and I will come across underpants. I know that two people in the family wear underpants like this, and that one of them is small and the other is a bit bigger. So are these underpants little or big? Suddenly, I realize that I cannot immediately tell. I cannot tell if these tiny purple underpants belong to my daughter or my wife. A particular kind of confusion, almost a whimsy.

'They're Leon's,' says Sarah brightly, looking over from where she's sitting, cross-legged on the sofa, controller in hand, leaning in to another car crash in Grand Theft Auto V, a video game about city-wide crime rampages which, like the movements of massive boats in the waters near our house, had become a primary means of escape for her since my diagnosis. 'I don't have any purple pants,' she adds. I briefly think of the underpants I first saw of hers on radiators in her old flat when we started going out, covered in pastel circles, friendly but intriguing: *somebody else's pants*. Then I return to sorting, and I think of the end of our driveway where I sort through recycling every other Thursday night, rummaging around in black boxes and dealing with wet cardboard and chunks of jagged glass.

Sorting is the kind of job I like now. It is simple and unambiguous and reeks of easy progress. And one Thursday night in March, winter finally giving way to spring as the evening light lingered and a cold breeze kept me company, I was puzzling, perhaps longer than I should have, over whether something was cardboard or tin, when I heard a posh 'Hello!' nearby and looked up to see a man standing in front of me.

This man was tall and elegant and beaming with the sheer happiness of having met me. His clothes were the casual clothes of a man who struggles when he is not wearing a suit: a dusty shirt tucked into flapping linen trousers, a neckcloth, a wide-brimmed hat in dirty cream. He looked sun-weathered even in March, but pleasantly so, stray pen strokes of black hair fringing his forehead. An aristocrat poet, perhaps, sinewy but arty. What was the right word? The right word was *statuesque*. Bryan Ferry. A. A. Gill.

'Hello,' I said, startled.

He carried a walking stick – not an aid for a limp, but a stick for cheery accompaniment while walking. 'I'm Michael,' he said. Or maybe, 'I'm Martin'; 'I'm Matthew.' He planted his feet firmly and swivelled his shoulders and torso and head to take in the scene, pink evening light turning to dark blue on the horizon. He was so practised in his movements he almost seemed animatronic. 'It's so beautiful here, isn't it? A special place.'

I looked around, and I suddenly realized that I agreed. 'It is beautiful,' I said. 'I love it here.'

He said a few more things, noted that he was glad to have met me and suggested, somehow, that he lived on the green too, just across the way, and that he had lived here for years. And then he wandered off to take in the evening. He was the kind of man who could do that: the kind of man who could take in an evening.

I saw him a few more times, spaced over a few weeks. We always had the same sort of chat. He was pleased to see me. He loved it here. *Wasn't it special?* It was only one afternoon in town as I mentioned him to Sarah that she informed me that this man was clearly a ghost.

'Only you see him? And he's dressed all Renaissance Faire?'

'More Man from Del Monte, but he was out of this era slightly.'

'And this weird chat: so pleased to see you, and isn't it lovely here, and doesn't it always stay the same?' She actually tutted at me. 'It is textbook ghost.' Putting a hand on my shoulder, she said, 'Tell me, was it suddenly a bit chilly around him?'

Sarah and ghosts: this is, remarkably, still the nurse part of her talking. The part that hates what she calls 'woo', and rejects contemporary society's boundless faith in the healing power of the avocado, the part of her that believes in vaccinations and finishing your course of antibiotics, is also linked to the part that opens a window on the ward when someone dies so their soul can fly like a singing bird.

I talked to a number of people about the ghost on the green. It had struck me at first as an unusual encounter but nothing more. Yet I did not trust my own reading of events after talking to Sarah. Results: a surprising number of people thought he was a ghost. A surprising number of people thought he was a hallucination.

Nobody thought he was real.

My dad thought he was a hallucination. 'But it seemed so convincing,' I said as we chatted one night on the phone.

'Hallucinations are sometimes convincing,' replied my dad, and told me a complex story about an episode in the 1980s, while working as a social worker, when he'd had to have committed a born-again Christian who had started power-mowing his lawn in the middle of the night because St Paul had asked him to.

'Did St Paul write him a letter?' I asked.

Dad ignored me. 'And think,' he said. 'If a person like you was going to hallucinate somebody, who would it be?'

'I don't know,' I said.

'I do,' said Dad. 'It would be a posh Englishman who's very friendly.'

After this, I spent an afternoon searching online, although, granted, as ever, I did not search very hard. Hallucinations caused by MS are rare, it seems. Exceedingly rare. But there are a few examples, sometimes ascribed to the drugs patients take rather than the disease itself, but generally reported by patients with advanced states of the disease.

Most of these cases were visual-release hallucinations, also known as Charles Bonnet syndrome, named for the Swiss naturalist who first described the condition in 1760. This type of hallucination – often of complex images: people, animals, cartoons – is exclusively the result of failing eyesight, which explains its link to MS, a disease in which eyesight is often impaired. Since my eyesight, that recent experience of diplopia aside, was no worse than normal, this suggests that my ghost on the green was neither a ghost nor a phantom of the mind. Besides, people with Charles Bonnet syndrome understand that the things they are seeing are hallucinations as they are happening. The people they see tend to be Lilliputian as well, and these tiny characters are unable to conduct conversations. They cannot speak at all.

Whenever the topic of hallucination and MS comes up online, however, I'll come across a stray comment that reminds people that the psychopathology of MS is itself under-explored territory.

In the end, regardless, I could not talk anybody around to my way of thinking. Nobody believed the man I had described was really there. 'If he is real,' said Dad, 'next time you see him, invite him in to meet Sarah.'

I still think the man on the green is real. I have always thought he was real, to be honest. I think he does exist and one day I will bump into him again and the whole thing will be concluded. And I also think that my willingness – at least to consider that he might be a ghost or a hallucination – is not MS. Not quite.

Instead, it is maybe something that has grown up alongside it. A cognitive slide I have allowed to take place, a hypochondriac grasping for some kind of mental disorder that I have felt should have arrived, and that, confusingly, sometimes genuinely has arrived. All of this is driven by a reduced confidence in what I am thinking and doing. At times, I am aware of a new thinness to my mental life, clearly visible in everything from my inability to follow conversations to the occasional total absence of an authorial voice in my own head. ('What kind of MS do you have?' patients sometimes ask other patients. 'Spinal MS? Blindness-and-paralysis MS?' Sometimes, I have narrative MS, a difficulty holding on to threads or creating new ones. I appreciate that this is probably one of the better forms of MS to have.) And so, even when I am feeling absolutely fine, I have taught myself that it is best to question the veracity of the things I am witnessing and the near-invisible glazes and tints of order I am applying to these things. Pulling all this apart is almost impossible, of course, like trying to turn the pages of a wet newspaper. And is it helpful to ceaselessly conduct this sort of self-examination?

At night, up late on my own around the time Sarah and I discussed the ghost on the green, I would sometimes have a moment of clarity, however. Exhausted by lack of sleep, I would sit, limbs burning, in a chair in the living room, and become fixed in time and space again, surrounded by my own house that ticked and settled in the darkness, back in the moment and suddenly capable of a rare kind of honesty. I saw, for example, that all the drama and exhilaration I was experiencing was still largely internal. I felt like I was living through a series of earthquakes: diplopia, neuralgia, fleeting periods of confusion. And yet I don't think any of this would have been apparent to anybody who knew me. I apologized more than usual, perhaps, and it was a rare day that didn't end with me sending an email to someone to explain something strange I had done earlier – but nobody else ever seemed to think I had been acting that strangely in the first place. Everything I felt going on was still going on inside, and maybe that meant I was managing everything.

And sometimes I was more than managing. Towards the end of March, I was discovering that there was another side to my particular experience of MS, a wild side that sometimes felt linked to the panic thrill of diagnosis, to the fact that my life had ceased to cruise and had entered what felt like a period of manic skidding. In between the double vision and the IKEA bed that I could not make, I was experiencing a rush of rogue positivity. I often became insanely chatty, filled with fidgeting questions: about medicine, about neurology and eventually about everything. I would go for a long, speedy walk around my neighbourhood – I told Sarah I was making the most of my legs while they still worked – and I would think: Why don't I know anything about magpies? Why don't I know the names of clouds? I took to carrying a notebook with me again, so many years after university, just so I could fill it with reminders to investigate all of the things I was suddenly curious about. Do magpies *really* collect silver? Is there really a kind of cloud called the undulatus, or was that just a dream? What does an undulatus look like? Who gets to name clouds?

And that line to Sarah, about using my legs while I still had them. That was not particularly sensitive, and it was typical of the insensitivity I was starting to express. This reminded me of someone – it did whenever I came back to earth, anyway. It reminded me of Phineas Gage, my handsome brother in neurology, who had become – what was the word? – *disinhibited*. I did not feel disinhibited when I was feeling good, but I did notice the quizzical, shocked looks I seemed to receive increasingly during conversations. They were the kinds of looks I might normally shoot at someone who had become disinhibited.

There were positives here, I told myself. MS was revealing not just that I had lived such a timid life. It was revealing that I had lived so much of that timid life on a kind of autopilot. In between moments of catastrophizing, I would sleepwalk, taking the same route to the bus each morning, sitting in the same seat on the bus, having the same kinds of thoughts as I stared out of the same window at the same view.

I was still trying to do all this, but in the presence of MS it was no longer entirely possible. There is that saying among neurologists: neurons that fire together wire together. It means that the synapses – those gaps between dendrites and axons, the inputs and outputs of neurons – that fire when messages make their way through the brain become stronger the more they are used, and therefore a constellation of synapses that has fired before is more likely to fire in the future. You get stuck in the same kind of behaviour by virtue of carrying out that kind of behaviour in the first place.

And suddenly, MS had come along and launched a handful of buckshot through all of that long-established wiring. That was my explanation, anyway. It certainly explained to me why kinks had started turning up in the ancient rituals of my life. Why I would look down at my hand on the bus and realize I was still holding a coffee cup from the house. Why I would leave home so many times over this period with my trousers undone. The patterns were breaking down and, trouser thing aside, maybe that wasn't such a disaster.

But I was scaring Sarah. She would return home from the store to find that I had surrounded Leon with teetering Lego palaces in her absence. Leon would be sitting in the middle of them all, bewildered by this sudden burst of construction. I would be equally bewildered to be told that this did not amount to *playing* with Leon. I also started to look odd, like I had been dressed by a malfunctioning robo-butler from the future, collars jagged, buttons done up wrong. When I looked after Leon, she started to look odd too. I often put her trousers on backwards.

I was learning the tidal break and pull of a relapsing and remitting disease – and all of the psychological clutter that comes with it so soon after diagnosis. And maybe, at first, this behaviour was the way the system bedded itself in. It marked the transition between being down, twitchy, achy, exhausted, sometimes mildly confused, and being up again, everything so sharp and bright that I felt like I could see every line in a stranger's face as I passed them in the street. Sometimes, just sometimes, I felt a tug at these moments, as if I wanted to stop the stranger and tell them all about it.

And this clarity, when it became decisiveness, was sometimes pretty handy. One night, in the bathroom, I felt water on my face and assumed that my trigeminal neuralgia had returned. In fact, there was another explanation: there was water on my face. A March shower had started outside, and now it was raining inside too, dripping through a fresh hole in the bathroom ceiling over by the pull cord for the light that I often struggled to find these days.

Raining indoors. Back before MS, this would have absolutely shattered me. I would have pictured the attic filling with a polluted midnight sea, the hatch above the living room buckling and then drowning Sarah, Leon and me, our bodies twisting in the thick, cloudy flood. I would have been dead and buried before I had even started to investigate. But now I just accepted that there was a hole in the roof somewhere and I needed to get it fixed, and there were probably people I could call who would do this. At most, we'd have to cut down on the weekly takeaway.

To me, this kind of basic objectivity felt like the blossoming of a new superpower, and it stayed with me long enough to survive several tradesmen telling me that the entire roof had to come off and be replaced, the 1930s tiles having been worn down by decades of coastal winds until they had the consistency of wet biscuit.

It even stayed with me through the three days it took to replace the roof, in which it became clear that the forces controlling the universe hated our bungalow with an unusual passion. Making tea for the man who was doing the work for us I managed to blow the electrics, which meant I had to look at the fuse box for the first time since we had moved in.

First I had to find it. The fuse box turned out to be a strange and ancient thing hidden at the back of a cupboard in the kitchen. I remembered having read about it in the survey we had commissioned, but I didn't remember the survey saying that it looked like the kind of technology you might have found on a U-boat in the Second World War. It was patched together with great ingenuity, and it was made of some sort of material that wasn't quite wood and wasn't quite plastic.

'Is that Bakelite?' I asked the man who was fixing our roof, and who had joined me for moral support.

'No idea,' said the man, leaning in for a closer look. 'But that fuse is actually foil from an old chocolate wrapper, and the one next to it is a rusty nail.'

At that, he started to inch away from the cupboard, and I called for an emergency electrician.

'I dealt with it,' I said to Sarah that night, as the last tiles were in place. 'I made it through the whole thing.' I breathed out theatrically. 'I'm feeling pretty good about things.' I paced around, shaking my limbs because of the tingling I felt, because of the energy I suddenly seemed to have inside me.

Sarah looked up from the nautical book she had been reading. The binoculars and vessel-tracking apps had given way to almanacs of the sea. (The night before she had awoken in the middle of the night, talking of narwhals.)

'I'm just reading about this thing old sailors used to get,' Sarah told me over the edge of her book. 'When they were on ships for long periods of time with no sign of land. They got this thing called calenture.' She picked up her computer and read aloud from an open tab: ' "A delirium occurring from heat stroke or fever, in which a stricken sailor pictures the sea as grassy meadows and wishes to dive overboard on to them." '

She looked at me evenly. 'I bet those sailors were feeling pretty good about things too.'

That night, in bed and feeling calmer, I told Sarah about my

growing worries regarding Leon, worries that had been with
me since I came back from seeing Brian. Worries that had been
bubbling away, wordlessly, never quite announcing themselves
openly because there was always something else – double
vision, euphoria, a leaking roof – to get in the way. 'I've realized that I worry for her about this one thing,' I said. 'I'm
worried that her life won't be perfect.'

I had reason to worry. She had come home from nursery that
day and announced, as clearly as she could, that the T-shirt I
had dressed her in that morning, a classic X-ray on black showing a ribcage, was a boy's T-shirt. We asked: 'Who told you
that?' And we told her that whoever did tell her was not correct. Too late, though. Sometimes, you are too late.

'Was her life ever going to be perfect?' asked Sarah, clearly frus-
trated with my inability to join the real world. 'Is anybody's?'

Somehow, I survived even this revelation, which normally
would have flattened me more than the roof. Maybe it was
euphoria. Maybe Sarah was right and I was close to climbing
over the side of the boat.

I made use of my new energy. I went back to trying to understand neurology, haphazard as my approach could be. I
discovered, to my dark delight, that fascinating, personality-
warping illnesses lay in every direction.

Every morning, before a day of playing games and writing
about them, of walking around with my legs aching and my
trousers undone, I would sit up in bed while Sarah and Leon
slept, and read about the brain going wrong. When Sarah
woke, I would draw her close to tell her about the worst I had
discovered. 'Can you believe,' I would start each morning. Can
you believe what? *Everything*.

'Can you believe that there is a neurological problem in
which people cannot see things when they are moving?'

'It's called akinetopsia,' said Sarah, checking Leon was sleeping happily. 'It was in an episode of *House*.'

Well. Can you believe that there's an illness where people are blind but are convinced that they can see? That there's an illness where people cannot stop rhyming the ends of sentences they hear? That there's an illness where people cannot forget anything?

'They can't forget anything?' asked Sarah.

'It's called hyperthymesia,' I said.

'Sounds handy,' said Sarah, who had spent all of the previous day looking for her phone.

'It's not that handy,' I said. 'Imagine your world filling up with references, with ancient sleights, clogged with ghosts everywhere you went.'

Sarah sat up and moved her hair around a bit. And then she stopped and looked at me and her eyes narrowed.

'What's going on?' she asked.

'I'm just reading,' I said. 'You told me to learn about neurology.'

'I didn't tell you to do anything,' she said. 'I said it might be good to learn about MS. Because you have it. This is something else. This is . . .'

'Butterfly collecting?' I asked. I had read that some neurologists call it butterfly collecting – all of the weird, fringe illnesses that make for a good diagnosis on *House*. The kind my sister and I, when we were young, would collect. We would pester my dad to tell us about the weirdest things he had encountered at work. Just the gruesome ones, Dad, we'd ask, filling out car journeys, trips to the supermarket, holidays. Just the ones where someone dies in an unspeakable way or has an aneurysm.

'Children are heartless,' I said, apropos of a memory I only then realized had been unfolding in my head. Sarah nodded, though. She understood the missing links in what we had been discussing.

'Is it possible,' she said, kicking back the duvet and preparing to rise, 'that you are so hung up on these different diagnoses because you're trying to change your own diagnosis?'

'Like I could change MS,' I said.

'Not the diagnosis you got from your neurologist,' Sarah said. She put a warm hand on my shoulder as she moved past me in the bed. 'The diagnosis you got from your dad afterwards. MS personality.'

Myelin, the Mysterious – and Misunderstood – Substance at the Heart of MS

It took a long time for me to see past Charcot. He dominated my tentative investigations into MS. His name was there on every Wikipedia page I turned to, and his portrait – stern nobility with the hint of something surprisingly gentle behind the eyes – stared out at me from the pages of the neurology books I flicked through in Brighton's Jubilee Library. Here was the man who had solved MS. For months I did not think much about what had come next.

But the study of MS did not end with Charcot, just as the more I looked, the more I realized it did not begin with him either. In the 1960s, the role that the immune system plays in MS was established, and over the last thirty years the first disease-modifying drugs have started to emerge for the relapsing-remitting form.

And then there is myelin, the white matter of the brain, which lies at the centre of MS. Over the last few decades, there has been a quiet revolution regarding our understanding of this strange substance.

Myelin was discovered by Rudolf Virchow, one of those improbably multifaceted figures the 1800s were so good at nurturing. Virchow was an anthropologist and a medical doctor, as well as a biologist, prehistorian, writer, editor, politician, and the man who, when challenged to a duel with Bismarck, proposed they fight by eating sausages, one of which had been poisoned. In the

eighteenth century, Luigi Galvani, who proved that
neurons sent their messages via electricity rather than
spirits, liquid or vibrations, which were all competing
theories of the day, was the first to pro pose there must
be a coating of some kind on these cells to insulate the
electricity. In 1854, Virchow found it, a fatty material
coiled around the axon. And yet, brilliant as Virchow
was, he thought this fatty material was inside the neuron
rather than outside it. And so myelin was given a name
derived from *muelos*, the Greek word for 'marrow'.

The role myelin plays in MS has been understood since
the early twentieth century, but the substance itself has
continued to be misinterpreted and perhaps underestimated. It is traditionally the grey matter, composed of
the dendrites and cell bodies of neurons, that gets the
credit for the exciting things the brain can do. In the
crackle of synapses, in the sudden puffs of neurotransmitters like serotonin, this bioelectrical circuitry somehow
creates both thought and action. Myelin merely binds
the axons.

Even here though, it is easy to misjudge the elegance of
this substance. The most common modern analogy for
myelin is that it fulfils the role of the plastic coating on an
electrical wire. But myelin doesn't just protect the axon
it's wrapped around, it actually increases the speed
at which electrical messages move through the axon.
Enormously.

The more you discover, the stranger the picture
becomes. You might assume that all axons in the central
nervous system are myelinated. In truth, most aren't. In
an area like the optic nerve, which requires the swiftest
of transmissions as it relays messages from the retina in
the eye to the visual cortex at the back of the brain,

almost all axons have a coating of myelin, but elsewhere it can be something of a rarity. Even in one of the supposed strongholds of white matter, the corpus callosum, a thick bundle of axons that connects the two hemispheres of the brain, only around 30 per cent of axons are myelinated.

The man who explained all this to me is Dr William Richardson, a research scientist studying neural development and plasticity – the brain's ability to reorganize itself by creating new neural connections throughout its life – at University College London. Richardson is one of a growing number of neuroscientists who think that myelin has been underappreciated in terms of the role it plays in the central nervous system. I went to visit him on a gusty winter's day to understand more.

Studies over the last few decades have indicated that myelin is more complex than we thought. Experts used to believe that myelination, the first surge of myelin through the central nervous system, was a process limited to the early years of child development, but we now know it often continues for far longer – sometimes well into adulthood. There are also signs that the brain might be able to choose to myelinate naked axons if it receives sufficient feedback that they are being heavily used.

This last point suggests to Richardson that myelin plays a role in learning – formerly thought to be the preserve of the grey matter. Richardson and his team created a series of mouse wheels with rungs removed at random, and then they set mice running on them. Typically, most mice would learn to run on these complex wheels very quickly, no matter how strange the arrangement of rungs became. And they did, unless they had been robbed of the ability to myelinate axons, in which case the learning process took much, much longer. The neurons still fired together and wired together, but nothing was coming along to then speed up the circuit.

I sat with Richardson for an hour or two in his office and watched his videos of mice running on their wheels. I had promised myself that I would not ask Richardson about the potential for future therapies that his work may hold. I don't know why I felt so strongly about this. Maybe simply being away from home with a tape recorder and notepad forced me to assume a more objective, dispassionate bearing. Maybe I felt that by asking him I would be bringing a third entity – my over-bearing disease – into the conversation.

In the end, of course, I gave in and asked him anyway. Richardson thought very carefully for a few seconds and then allowed that it was possible that the cells scattered through the brain that seem to be monitoring axon use might one day be convinced to remyelinate after damage from disease. He mused that it might be beneficial for MS patients simply to keep learning new things.

That last thought has stayed with me. It seems not just wise and optimistic but an idea I can actually do some-thing with. Maybe sitting down at the piano is a meaningful form of therapy. Maybe learning Spanish with an audiobook could help a little bit. Maybe, when Leon comes to me tangled up with another of English's endless irregular verbs, I should look up why this particu-lar verb is irregular in the first place, and in doing so I might be aiding both of us in some tiny but happy way.

7. Hyde

On the coast road, the sky and sea are two kinds of silver meeting; the wind-farm rigs hover on the horizon, huge but flimsy. Here, I am thinking, is a dangerous day. For the last few miles I have been looking for signs and signals, augurs of the hours to come. In other words, I am on my way to a neurology appointment.

It's a routine appointment in late March, and I have been enjoying the prospect of seeing Dr Quill again. As I brushed crumbs from my shirt a few hours earlier and even tucked it in, I glimpsed Sarah smirking at me from the bed, knowing that I was just seconds from staring in the mirror and asking: 'Does this *work*?'

But at the outpatients unit I find that Dr Quill is passing me over, just for the day – not to Koenig, my MS specialist, but to yet another new neurologist. She is very tall and very young with bright eyes and a brisk, emphatic handshake. She tells me she is delighted to meet me. She tells me that she has seen my brain scans. She leads me into a room with a handful of monitors, all of which depict cross-sections of a brain. The silvery lines of an MRI image make the bones of the skull shimmer, while the brain within is a grainy shadow, as if buried beneath storms.

So it is Wednesday, and for the first time in my life I am staring at my brain. I am sitting in a crumbling Victorian room in a crumbling Victorian building, and I can see my brain right there on the screen in front of me. Actually it's on several screens in front of me: different sections, different angles, different resolutions. All told, there is plenty of my brain to go around.

I can meddle with it, to a certain extent. I can take the mouse – this is allowed but not encouraged – and spin the scroll wheel. And then, with that peculiar corrugated chug, I suddenly fly through this ugly grey mass, from the bottom, with its arresting and grim hint of a lamb shank, to the top, a rumpled plateau enlivened by the occasional dark river of vein or artery.

It does not look like a pleasant place to visit. But visiting is an idiotic thought. It strikes me suddenly: this is where I live. I have spent my whole life inside this gritty, ghostly lump, even if it has taken thirty-six years and a certain degree of catastrophe to lead me to this lofty perspective. It feels, in a giddy sort of way, like escape, but I know that I have not escaped. I am still in there. My brain is still in there. My brain is looking at my brain. If I'm honest, it is thinking: Is this it?

I tell myself: Listen, as far as we know, the human brain is the single most complex thing in the entire universe.

Yes, yes. But you'd think it would make a more striking first impression. Even so, everything I have seen, everything I have ever thought, is captured on the screens in front of me somewhere, in some wordless form.

This feels so wrong. To be inside a brain and looking at it at the same time. And for all my explorations, I realize that I am still a tourist at best. I have no real idea what I'm seeing. I don't know what the various lumps depicted on the scans do, and whether the dark spots are benign or a cause for concern. I don't know if the veins I see rambling over the surfaces are actually veins at all, and I don't know if I'm looking at the grey matter or the white.

Where are the landmarks I have read about? Where is the amygdala, the engine of fear? Where are the hippocampuses, left and right, and is that even the right plural? Where are the *neurons*, the machinery of thought, grasping and inquisitive, but also spectral, delicate, and nothing like any machine I know of?

The drama of MS is almost impossible to spot. I expect raging white bursts of light – forest fires burning in the neurogenic darkness. Instead, my new neurologist points out scattered patches of fine mist. That's where the trouble is, apparently. That is MS. It doesn't seem very dramatic at all – until, when I stumble home later, I suddenly understand that the mist appeared to be scattered in a number of different locations.

I can't remember what I have been brought here to discuss. I can't remember much of what I am told over the course of our fifteen-minute consultation. I'm pretty sure another MRI is mentioned, though – scheduled for the end of the year, to monitor the drugs I am taking.

One other thing: I remember the neurologist suddenly asking, on the way out, if I've fully grasped what I've just seen. I must have betrayed myself somehow, a twitch or a certain blankness. She is asking, I think, in a kind, concealed way, if she showed me too much.

Too much? That white mist, I want to say, that ghostly landscape, it is too little. It is all too little.

When Sarah asked how my appointment had gone, I mumbled something cheerful and fake and shut the door to the spare room. I had taken the day off work for the scan, and so I spent the entire afternoon in there alone, which amounts to an aggressive act in a marriage like ours. I was busy at least, carefully rejecting everything that I had seen. Faced with something I could probably understand with a bit of work, I turned away from it.

It was hard work, this rejection. Luckily, in the days that

followed I had help. I had the whole universe. The next morning at work, someone emailed around a little video of Laniakea,
Hawaiian for 'immeasurable heaven', the galaxy supercluster
that the Milky Way forms a tiny, truly insignificant part of.
Galaxy superclusters are the largest objects in the entire universe. Recent changes in thinking about these massive objects
have led to alterations in the way they are demarcated, and
within the number-juggling and the tracking of swift, silent
celestial bodies, Laniakea had been discovered, vast yet delicate, its galaxies flowing together like cars on an LA highway,
drawn towards an area of space known as the Great Attractor.
On their way, they formed huge spectral filaments picked out
in gold in the video. Our supercluster, one of many millions,
looked so fragile, a massive, wind-blown feather, arcing and
trilling through space, unknown and unseeable until explorers
had come along with the right means of revealing it.

I could not watch this video without starting to cry. There is
no time, I thought. That's what Laniakea tells us. There is no
time for a thing this big. Even if we started today, even if we
started at the beginning of time itself, there is not enough time
to get a sense of what a thing like this means, what it is truly
like, what it is capable of producing. Its full capability for wonder is unknowable, and cannot be realized. It is all a waste.

My brain, in comparison, the measly brain I had seen on the
screens at the hospital, started to diminish in its power, which
had been, for the last twenty-four hours, the power to make me
feel sick and stupid. 'It looks kind of like a brain?' Dan, a colleague, said, leaning over my shoulder as we watched Laniakea
twisting back and forth on my monitor. 'No,' I said, with a little too much force. 'It looks like a feather.' My tone announced
that the conversation was over, and Dan went back to his desk.
With him gone, I opened a document to write something about
video games, found that I was freshly wordless, and opted for

interview transcription instead, to give the blinking cursor on my screen something to do.

I had my first symptoms in January 2014 and it was now late March 2015; I was well into my second year of MS. How was I doing? I was doing very badly. But I often told myself I was doing very well. As a result, for much of the first half of 2015 I was a monster.

Nobody tells you that you will know the bad times by the seemingly good times that accompany them. I spent my early days with MS floating back and forth between a state of absolute confusion and a state of absolute certainty, thinking that I had cracked it, that I finally understood what MS was and what it meant for me.

These opposing sensations – the fog of complete bewilderment, the toxic Zen of total comprehension – refused to maintain a polite distance. They would flow together, cancelling each other out. I would entirely forget one state as I raced into its equal, its opposite, zipping back and forth in days, sometimes mere hours. Opposing ways of being lost. And the worst of these, in retrospect, was the state in which I did not feel lost at all.

One night in May I went out for a quick post-work drink with people from the office. Around this time, in my memory, at least, I was frequently stumbling over sentences – a clumsiness in my speech probably powered by a growing fatigue – and at work I was often silent, afraid to say a word in case someone noticed what a mess I was and sent me home.

But I was also, sadly, this idiot going out for a drink with his friends, someone who spoke, more or less, in a clear voice, and who rambled on with a grotesque smugness about all the things that MS had taught him about the world. Someone who seemed firmly in charge of his own life and willing, even, to tell everyone what they should be doing with theirs. This is not someone

I would want to be stuck in a lift with. And yet, somehow, it was me. It was me, speaking, from a position of obvious ignorance, of ugly, arriviste certainty, on behalf of everyone with MS.

I was a surprisingly eloquent idiot that evening, banging on about my grand unified theory of MS, about how it was all about mindfulness, about living in the moment because the future was in doubt while the present was a concrete certainty that could be enjoyed, that *had* to be enjoyed. Nobody had asked me, but still I spoke at length about my world – or rather, I offered a view on to it in which everything was very carefully arranged to make me look excellent. The drugs I'm on are working, I explained, hinting that the illness was held in neat didactic balance with the rest of my life. And yes, in some ways – look! – MS is even helping me to be a better person.

I believed this at the time, or I wanted to. I wanted this approach I had found, this helpful, euphoric way of looking at the world, to expand, panoramically, until it explained everything I might come up against. Living in the moment!

But I forgot things. I forgot, for example, that it is not all about me. Other people have been dragged along on this ride with me, and they may need me to be able to step outside of the moment I am bravely enjoying so much and picture the future every now and then. And beyond that, the ignorance and arrogance: I was discussing strategies for handling a disease that, at the time, I had only just met. What of those who had known MS a long time? Would I have spoken so freely with them, if I could bear to meet them? Would they be impressed by my chirpy approach to tackling the disease we all faced?

My monologue that evening built to the most insane crescendo, in which I appeared to speak on behalf of my people. And my people, astonishingly, were suddenly people with disabilities in general. I was acting like the Malcolm X of people with disabilities, even though, if I had given it a moment's thought, I was not yet disabled, and am still not yet disabled. Even though I had not really considered what it meant to wake up every day disabled in even the smallest way. Even though I had not considered the vital difference between realizing that, one day, I might be disabled through MS, and experiencing an entire lifetime of being treated the way people with disabilities are often treated.

'People need to see people like me,' I said to my colleagues, as if my disease were in any way visible to most of the people I passed on the street. There was anger here – maybe that morning I had to stand on a packed bus for five minutes while I secretly, invisibly, had MS the whole time. And there was shame too. Shame about the fact that I had spent the last thirty years letting people with disabilities iris out in my peripheral vision. I must have done this, because Brighton suddenly seemed freshly filled with them. This was no sudden epidemic. These people had simply become visible again.

I accept that all of this is me. The egomania. The blinkered certainty. Even the feeling that MS had boosted me to a higher level of awareness and perspective, rather than merely facilitated access to a new and rarefied tier of triteness and self-involvement. This person was me, and is me.

Still, he had his grim uses. He proved that there is a sense of progress in decline. Nobody tells you about this either.

Sometimes, like that evening in the bar, I could speak clearly, even if I wasn't always saying things worth listening to. Sometimes, over the same period, I could struggle with even the simplest words. Strange. And deeply untypical for early MS. I am still puzzling over it.

In April I picked up a stutter that started out as an object of interest and steadily became maddening. Sentences suddenly exhausted me, the way a trip into town had started to exhaust me, the very thought of it as wearying as the act of walking. Some days I was fine; on other days, sentences appeared like dusty roads, baked by the sun, stretching into the distance with so much opportunity for incident – potholes, collisions, fainting – before I reached the end.

Is this the thought process of a stutterer? I didn't know, but even then I suspected it wasn't. Do stutters come and go the way this one did, dropping by for fifteen minutes, for an hour? Do you even get stutters with MS? I didn't know. As soon as the stutter was at full force – and at full force it was bad enough that I had to cancel phone interviews for work – I began to doubt how real it was. As words grew harder to finish, I wondered if I was just winding myself up and creating phantoms for myself, finding reasons not to engage. Allan Ropper is an American neurologist who has written a wonderfully pulpy book about his life on the neurology ward of a teaching hospital in Boston. It has an entire chapter on phantoms, false positives, and people who are outright faking. I never felt like I was faking anything, but to my shame my stutter went away when I read that chapter. It scurried away, exposed. The problem with having a disease that's all in your head is that there are other things in your head at the same time.

To make things worse, I was starting to lose the odd word by itself. Parts of my vocabulary were flickering in and out of existence, as if my sentences were being fed rattling through some kind of cognitive hole punch. If it was late in the day, or if I was consumed by some worry or preoccupation, I might reach for words and find that some of them weren't there any more. Everyone knows a little of this experience, I think, but it was happening to me with annoying regularity – so much in fact that it broke into the realm of gesture, and I started to do a little windmill motion with my right hand to suggest to whoever I was speaking that I was still going to finish my thought.

There were other ways of coping. At work, I typed more and tried to speak less. Out with friends, I would settle on the periphery of a conversation, permanently exhausted. Only at home did I still try to make myself understood all the time.

It wasn't always just words. At some point in summer I was talking to a builder on the phone. Another part of my house was falling down – the host rejecting yet another graft. The builder asked for my phone number. I thought about it. I thought about it some more. I felt worryingly serene. 'I'm sorry,' I said, 'I can't remember.' He asked for my address. 'I'm sorry,' I laughed. 'I can't remember that either.'

And this was fine.

Honestly, it really was fine. Initially I felt pretty delirious about how fine it was. Maybe, I told myself after I had hung up from the builder, I have been a slave to memory for too long. I liked the sound of that, the pomposity of it: *a slave to memory for too long.* When I was a child, I would spend hours trying to remember all the words to 'Dover Beach', by Matthew Arnold, only because we lived quite close to Dover and my mother loved Arnold, and it would drive her nuts if I started quoting the poem in a silly voice whenever we drove past the seafront in her Morris Traveller. I had most of it down pretty well, but I got hung up on 'melancholy, long, withdrawing roar', which always seemed to bubble up as 'melancholy, dark, departing roar', allowing Mum a gap in which to point out my mistake. That used to drive *me* nuts, and then I'd drive myself nuts again trying to somehow force the phrase into my brain correctly. A thing I had invented to send my dear old mother crazy had backfired elegantly.

Nowadays, it wouldn't have. Nowadays, I just didn't care. I was past remembering – past remembering even Matthew Arnold, who had said some things worth keeping close about the various iniquities of time and of health.

'The sea is calm tonight.' Even the simplest, most tangible of everyday things sometimes required elaborate workarounds. I described a shower head as a speaker that water comes out of. When I forgot the word *windowsill*, I described it as the little pavement that lies next to the glass. I would say that Leon's funnel or beak needed cleaning when I meant her mouth, and in the rush to write something down on a calendar, I would instead forget calendars themselves, and I would ask Sarah for an alphabet of months.

And at first it was all so liberating. It was liberating to be able to say, 'I don't know,' and move on, and to have the perfect excuse too. MS, at its heart in the very early days, when you take away the nerve pain, the buzzes, the pops, the intricate unfurling of a new symptom, seemed both an agent of change and an excuse for coping with that change in any manner I wanted – and at the expense of almost everything else. On the good days, it was carte blanche for forgetting everything, and not caring about any of it.

But it was not liberating for ever. I sense now that the enjoyment I'd taken in forgetting is not the work of MS, neither is the speed at which I allowed myself to give up on trying to remember what I had forgotten. These aren't clinical symptoms, perhaps. No, in my case these symptoms feel worse than that. They're part of what I feared at first and then forgot to fear – that MS could be such a wonderful, powerful all-purpose excuse I might invoke it a little too often. Without proper care and attention, the very idea of it might become a factor in a slow, steady retreat from the world – until one day I was so far back that I wouldn't hear its melancholic, dark, departing roar any more.

Can you grieve for yourself? I asked myself one day. I was reading Joan Didion's *The Year of Magical Thinking*. Didion has MS, but this book focuses on other concerns. It describes the year that followed the sudden death of her husband, and in grief, she suggests, we experience strange things. Things that feel, to me, a lot like certain symptoms I had associated with neurology. Concentration is lost. Cognitive ability is reduced. Word blindness, blundering, the forgetting of one's own phone number. So was this grief in the mix? Can you grieve for yourself? I asked this, and heard the answer: yes.

Is that MS, with the vanishing words? Anomic aphasia, or a problem with word retrieval, is caused by damage to the parietal or temporal lobes. It has been seen in MS often, and it is a common accompaniment to many kinds of brain injury. So it's possible. Is it fatigue? The sheer stress of diagnosis? Or is it a mix of that along with some subconscious decision that my frequently invisible disease needed a means of announcing itself, and that it should have a voice, even if it was found by poking holes in my own?

In time, I came to think of MS — and the cruelties, sometimes self-inflicted, that I brought with it — as a hollowing out of the parts of me that I liked, and that made me who I thought I was. It was hard to spot, however, because hollowing is internal, and the mask often remained in place, like the jagged smile on a Halloween pumpkin. (*Hollowing* — it is a word, I discovered recently with a weird flush of something like pride, that Oliver Sacks sometimes uses for his patients.) I was left with an empty, rattling head, too muddled to think, a person who stumbles into door frames and mutters at his own daughter.

But only sometimes. One day tripping over words, the next day speaking perfectly clearly. So add unpredictability to the mix.

And maybe the muttering part of this person had its own name. I had reread *Dr Jekyll and Mr Hyde* in the sweet, sleepy days shortly after Leon was born. It had stayed with me, as it always does, but this time there had been something new about the way it lingered in my mind.

I have often found myself thinking of Robert Louis Stevenson as I have become ill. He was always a favourite, and I had also been struck by something I discovered rereading a recent biography. Stevenson was a 'professional sickist', at the mercy of various lung illnesses. The biography I read suggested that it's possible that Stevenson was a great writer in part because of these illnesses, rather than despite them. Maybe the debilitating slumps he experienced throughout his life somehow forced him towards bursts of bright action when he was well. Disease told him that time was short and energy was to be treasured, that his life was a tiny chunk of flaming magnesium.

But if I believed that, I felt I had to confront the broader picture too. Now, I returned to *Hyde* once again, reading it across a period of several evenings as Leon sat in my lap and flicked the edges of my book, enjoying the sound and the sense of involvement, and the sudden gust of air the pages made.

Mr Hyde is the most famous invention of anyone with a relapsing disease, and perhaps, when Stevenson first dreamed him up, he was not only thinking of the 'hidden self' that was such a popular theory in repressed Victorian society. Perhaps he was also confronting the manner in which a disease that comes and goes plays a special kind of havoc with a person's identity. All of that seemed captured in *Dr Jekyll and Mr Hyde*, but transformed, reworked, almost concealed. Stevenson wrote in vivid bursts and relapsed viciously – days and weeks in bed staring at the ceiling, or playing with his son-in-law's tin soldiers on the rug, rumpled to look like a mythical landscape. These instances have the rhythm of Jekyll's sudden transformations, although morality has crept in somewhere to complicate everything. Still, the tidal shift is visible, the ebbing process that takes Jekyll from apparently decent Victorian to stomping beast, from dishonest refinement to a kind of honest horror.

I wondered suddenly about my own back-and-forth relapses: how they change me. The symptoms, but also the things I alone was bringing to them, the way I was letting MS chip away at my patience while I replaced it with self-pity and bitterness. Is this the MS personality that Dad mentioned? Or is this just me?

I wouldn't be the first neurological patient to feel that there are two people inside my head – and that I don't like one of them. And it's Leon who makes me worry about Hyde the most. My Hyde is a tricky one, quietly – and invisibly – trading places with me when the moment takes him. Late spring, the sun surprisingly harsh, I seemed to be all relapse. I was often too exhausted and twitchy to look after Leon properly on the days I had her by myself, the Saturdays and Sundays when Sarah had to take a weekend shift at work. *Peppa Pig* became a shameful accomplice in these moments: a way of giving in and just letting Leon watch television while I creaked and murmured on the sofa, sounding out one ache after another. I grew snappy with her, and I would rather lounge about than play.

But I still listened to her. I love Leon's words. I have loved almost all of them, at every stage. She has made me see the power of simple words, and she has made me see that clumsiness and eloquence can exist in a single sentence, like the other day, when we were listening to the radio, and she suddenly turned, eyes wet with happy tears, to say: 'There is much music inside me.'

There are some words of hers I hate, however, and none more than the word she uses when I ask how she is feeling. She doesn't say *fine*, or *okay*, or *happy*, *grumpy*, *angry*, *sad*. She says:

Better. She says she is feeling better even if she hasn't been ill. It is an answer that has management imprinted on it – an answer that pre-emptively counters a parent's fretting and neuroses. It is an answer that tries to create a little space when love becomes worry and worry grows claustrophobic and bullying.

Let me take you into the worst of it. It is a sunny Saturday in May but the sun is oppressive and startling. Inside, it seems that the heating has been left on, but the radiators are cold when I touch them. I sense a churning through the floorboards, rising up through my legs and spine and settling behind my eyes. But the dishwasher is silent – I have checked – and the washing machine is not spinning. The house looks terrible, cups perched on bookcases, cat hair and grit sticking to my feet. *Peppa Pig* is on the television, of course, and Sarah is out at work.

It is the dangerous low point of the afternoon. I am clogged with self-pity and the start of a cold. It all seems so impossibly lengthy and arduous. Arms aching, legs aching, palms prickling and fingers tingling, I see my life with MS – my life as a failing parent, as an incomprehensible, moody idiot – reaching off into the distance like one of the endless sentences I am currently struggling with, each thought's transition into words exhausting. I should do something. What would a good parent do? They would take their child out into the sun somewhere. I can imagine a park, a library, a pool of calm in the city. I can imagine making it that far.

I find Leon in the nursery, arranging dolls. 'Let's go out!' I say. She jumps up and starts to hop on the spot with sheer energy. Let's get rid of some of that, I think, as I check there are nappies, spare clothes, snacks in a bag, as I track back to the porch to prime the pushchair and brush out the crumbs.

Then I lose myself in fiddling with a loose screw on the pushchair. It seems I fiddle with it for several minutes. When I emerge from this fixing trance, it strikes me that a longish time has passed. 'Where are you, Leon?' I ask. I walk back into the living room.

She is not ready to go yet. She's laying her summer jacket on the floor.

I check my phone. The bus is leaving soon. I haven't got a ticket, so I fumble through the purchase. 'We have to get going, darling,' I say, with an edge rising in my voice. She is still messing with her jacket, turning it inside out, stretching out the arms, smoothing it.

My pin for the bus app is wrong. I fumble with it some more, typing it in again. My staticky hands are useless. Again. One last chance before I'm locked out. Five minutes until the bus comes, and then an hour's wait for the next one.

I look up, ticket purchased. Why is the heating still on? Why is Leon still screwing around with her jacket, brushing it out on the floor, arranging it to some strange design when the bus is almost here? Why is she even thinking of wearing a jacket on a day like today?

Out of nowhere, I am furious. No build-up, I yell: 'LEON, PUT THAT FUCKING JACKET ON!'

And I see it all unfold. She is caught in a movement as I yell at her, already committed. And the movement is beautiful. She is gripping the ends of the arms of the jacket with a dexterity and grace I did not know she possessed. She is flipping the jacket up and over her head so that somehow it arranges itself on her like a magic trick, arms in the right holes, sleeves sliding into place, jacket falling around her exactly as it should. This is what the smoothing out was for. She was priming the jacket for this piece of bright wonder.

And now that the moment is used up, the careful pre-planned cycle has fired, so she is able to register what I have said. Her proud smile wobbles, something inside her face, her resolve, that splinter of happy defiance that I now realize is the absolute core of my astonishing daughter, starts to shudder. And she cries and hides her face. She thought I would be proud of her, delighted at what a big clever girl she is becoming.

When Leon finally turns back to me, I am crying too. Terrible thing. The wordless trauma of being young and expecting order in all the important elements, and then seeing your mother or father crying. This impossible sight, this inversion, and yet here it is.

The truth is, my optimism has relapses.

In the books and the pamphlets they talk of a 'drunk feeling' with MS, the sudden transition from being sober to being absolutely ploughed, everything around you amusingly incoherent. And I definitely get that. I know what it's like to walk down a street, finding each advertisement I pass more obliquely amusing than the last.

But I also get a consumed feeling. A strange state to be in, as if the conscious part of me – the me who is always busy talking to me about what is going on – has somehow slipped deeper inside and I am staring up at the world from the bottom of a dark red well. Suddenly I am subtly removed from things, witnessing my own movements with a certain professional distance.

LEON, PUT THAT FUCKING JACKET ON. I am not claiming that this took place in the consumed state. I wish it had. Look at it, though. Bare coherence. No punctuation can fix the ugliness of that sentence, the raggedness, the brutal curtness of it. The words are maybe a tenth of the toxic cargo that is being communicated. The doll, Poppy, face down against the skirting board again. Upside down, it is all upside down.

It reminds me of the terrible, inadequate men my mum accidentally filled some of our childhood with, my sisters and me, when Dad had gone. A drunken gardener. An irritable military type who loved vampire movies. A man or two from here and there – and always, underneath the naff variables, the same man.

I don't want to be that man. I worried about him a lot when Sarah was pregnant, in between worrying about the house and worrying about every other thing in the world, of course. I woke one night and my fears had organized themselves to form a neat sentence: *I don't want to be another adult who isn't grown-up enough to have a child in their lives.* And I see now, bad as MS is, gentle as I have it so far, that I cannot blame it for everything. If I fail with Leon, I will be the one failing. I don't even think that MS would count as an accessory.

An accessory. The language of the courts. Your own parents go on trial the day your first child is born. With luck, you go on trial shortly afterwards.

At least I can see it, I tell myself for days after I have shouted at Leon. At least I can see it. I don't want my daughter raised by Hyde. I don't want my daughter raised by a man who cannot see that Hyde is a part of him, and that he must control all parts of himself.

That summer I was starting to realize that while my MS could always get worse, my handling of it could not. I was manic and unpredictable at work and at home, wordless one minute and ranting about optimism the next. I was delighted to get to the end of each day without having upset myself, but I often neglected to notice how much I had upset the people around me.

Something had to change. And then all of a sudden it did. I can still remember the moment.

It was the day I decided I was going blind.

And this, it so happened, was the day after I had been out to a costume party. A friend of mine always throws a big

Halloween party, and we always dress up and attend. I took Leon to her first when she was a couple of months old. I have a photograph of her, tiny and dressed in a skeleton onesie, half asleep in the arms of a friend, done up as Ronald McDonald. That would have been Halloween 2013. Halloween 2014 was derailed by scheduling problems, so it was shunted to the summer of 2015. Sarah was tired that night and wanted to stay in with Leon. I was manic, so I went to the party, but I had to throw together a costume from stuff that I found in the kitchen at the last minute. No problem, though: I had a brilliant idea. All I needed was a cardboard tube, tin foil to cover it in, and an elastic band to hold it in place on my head.

'You're going as Phineas Gage,' Sarah observed as I collected my keys. It wasn't a question, and I sensed something brittle behind the words. Then she shut the door on me and I wandered to the bus, a cardboard tamping iron leaning drunkenly out of my forehead. I was laughing to myself as I went, off for an evening of making everyone who knew me deeply uncomfortable.

I didn't drink, because I was still unsure as to how Pimm's would mesh with my new medication. I got the bus home early in the end, slipping into bed next to Sarah and Leon, and then I awoke before everyone else the next morning. In the creamy dawn light of a perfect June day I noticed it was starting. Blindness.

I had been waiting to go blind – waiting not with panic, as I gather that the blindness you get with MS does not last, or at least not often. Waiting instead with a kind of quiet interest. What would it be like to be blind?

It was like this: when I opened my eyes I saw a grey spot, a shifting, agitated scribble written in soft pencil and dancing just off the centre of my vision. I closed both eyes but it remained in place when I opened them again.

Calmly I reached for my phone and composed an email to an editor colleague. *I may need a few days off work*, I typed. *I think I am going to be blind for a bit.*

Such dangerous complacency. *I think I am going to be blind for a bit.* Maybe this is what it's like sometimes, I told myself, to have MS in the early years of the twenty-first century. I wrote three or four emails, and I planned things. What to do about the house, about getting Leon to childcare, about the shopping, the bins, a present for a friend's birthday. And then I went back to sleep.

The blindness did not arrive – the scribble had faded by midday, but by then I had broadcast my heroic ambivalence towards blindness loudly to Sarah and Leon.

I think sometimes that early MS is a sort of tasting menu of neurological disease. It is also a tasting menu of life, of all the experiences that can make up a life, or many lives. I sample so many things and then move on. The trick, though, is to engage – even with the awful stuff. To engage, to own it, to experience the fear and the horror and the feeling small and unfortunate. Even with the awful stuff, even as you hope, occasionally with genuine panic, that it will soon end. Had I engaged with this in any way? Or had I just made a grim theatre of my competence?

'If I'm not blind, I should probably go to work,' I said to Sarah around lunchtime. I went hunting for my keys and, when I came back, I saw that Sarah was crying. She was watching Leon play on the carpet, and she was sobbing, silently, with no intention of alerting me to it. This was not theatre. It never is. She would have let me disappear off to work like this.

I sat beside her. She did not go out of her way to make room for me. I awkwardly put an arm around her. 'It's fine,' I said. 'It didn't happen.'

'How can you do all this?' she said. 'How can you saunter from one catastrophe to the next? How can you walk around like you're acing it? How can you quietly plan for blindness? How can you go to a party dressed like you've got a bar through your head and expect people to be delighted?'

'I'm dealing with it,' I said. 'We're dealing with it. I'm just deep inside it at the moment.'

'You're not, though,' she said, eyes narrowed by tears. 'You never are. You're above it. You're always somewhere above it all, floating around. You're explaining it away, coping with it in some stupid fashion that nobody else understands, proving that it's nothing to worry about, when it is. It is something to worry about.'

She explained to me what she had witnessed that morning. She explained that it is an affront to approach blindness with calm. You should acknowledge it as a terror, a thing that has ruined people's lives.

And at the heart of my response to blindness, she detected a coping mechanism gone insidiously wrong: a means of denial that looks like clear-eyed acceptance and the processing of trauma.

'So would it have been better if I'd panicked?' I asked.

She didn't answer me. Instead she looked away, and said: 'This neurology jag you're on. It started as a means of understanding the disease.' I stared blankly at Leon on the carpet as she spoke. 'But the more you've read, the more it's become something else. It's become a way of distancing yourself from the reality of this situation, and the reality is simple.

'You are not a doctor,' Sarah said. 'You are a patient. You have a brain, and it is going wrong, and while that is exciting and inspiring, you need to confront the fact that it is also a disaster, to step away from the theory and see what is happening. And then we need to work out what kind of life we can lead now that this disaster is here.'

★

The question Sarah finally posed was not going to be easy to answer: what does our life look like now if we try to put MS in some kind of wider context?

We decided to find out, and instead of hunting for an immediate answer, for a handful of quiet months we simply lived very tentatively together, trying to tempt a sense of normality back to our lives, as if we were leaving food out each night for a cat that had just taken off one day.

It was wonderfully undramatic. We fixed stuff around the house. We bought Leon new clothes as she grew out of her old ones, and we decided which tiny trousers and T-shirts to pass on to other parents and which we could not be without.

In search of small things to focus on, I started to learn how to complete cryptic crosswords. A throwaway distraction, perhaps, but one that gave me vital moments of glinting victory every lunchtime at work, and would eventually stretch to fill an entire Sunday afternoon, Sarah and I pitching clues and solutions through the house, as I ploddingly moved from solving the odd line here and there to attempting an entire grid.

I saw Jennifer, my MS nurse, more often than I had before, regular meetings in the windowless room with the model of the femur on the table between us as we picked over the concerns that intrude every so often into the life of someone who has MS but who also has the lingering suspicion that they are getting MS wrong. That was a big part of the problem, I discovered. I felt I was getting MS wrong. I would lurch back and forth between conflicting paranoias: that I had a much more severe form of the disease, or even a different disease entirely, or that I had no disease at all and was simply making trouble for everyone for no reason.

One day Jennifer said to me that MS is not like breaking an ankle. She said that the very nature of it requires a degree of interpretation, and at the beginning that can be overwhelming.

She made it clear to me that I would come to understand it all, that I would get to a point where I could recognize the phantoms – the fears and compensations and overreactions – and also recognize the points at which the disease was genuinely advancing.

Language again: with Jennifer, more than anything, I was learning how to interrogate my illness, how to draw a new symptom into the light and give it context. I was now truly learning what she had told me in our first meeting: that I was the first and the only person to have this form of MS, because each form of MS is a one-off. I was learning to recognize my new self.

I had ranted about mindfulness at length before, but with Jennifer's help, language revealed that, while the future with MS is frightening, for me it really does play most of its tricks in the absolute present. For me, MS is an attack on the moment itself, on my instantaneous processing of the moment. It is an adverbial disease, belonging to that same liminal, mediating area that adverbs operate within. Adverbs are an attempt to interrupt a thought or action as it is happening, and nuance the understanding of that thought or action in some way. This is where MS strikes, where it undermines: when I am trying to make a bed, or get a baby ready for her bath.

My illness itself was changing throughout this period. The maddening cognitive tricks seemed to be retreating and my speech was improving, while my physical symptoms became clearer and more pronounced. An ache in my calves spread to my thighs, to my groin; I needed to rest every half hour or so if we headed into town. I got a headache most evenings which felt like a metal band was tightening around the top of my skull, and in the morning I would discover that I had been gripping my hands so fiercely during the night that my finger-nails had left angry little dents in my palms. The idea that I might ever feel fraudulent about MS became hilarious to me. Even when MS seemed nearly silent, I would have a strange, warming, internal tremor that gave my voice a little quaver, and at its worst, any kind of overexertion would make me feel like thin rods of metal had been pushed down through my arms and legs, down through the pelvis and the inside of my thighs, as if someone had straightened a metal coat hanger and slid it into me. One afternoon in London, visiting the Courtauld, I saw one of Degas's ballerina bronzes, and moving in close noticed part of her wire frame protruding through an elbow. I laughed out loud. Recognition.

Largely, I managed to take these things as they were: my MS was coming into focus, and I refrained from trying to make any more sense of it than that. I had the occasional lapse into florid certainty and grand proclamations of the kind I had shared with my work colleagues when we went out for a drink, but only when someone was stupid enough to ask how I was *really* doing. Most of the time, MS was something private and quiet.

Throughout all this, Leon dazzled me. Leon, whose eruption of new tricks was far more interesting than anything my body could come up with. She was growing so quickly again. Each new day there seemed to be more of her – longer limbs, longer hair, rounder cheeks. And there was more to her mind too. I could say that this was because of the dendrites tangled on top of her neurons, stretching out their arms as if waking and yawning. But why phrase it like that? Why give neurology absolutely everything? Leon had made new connections, had uncovered new abilities. She had discovered a new appetite for experience.

One month it was sentences. 'Me eating an apple, Dadda.' And she was. The next month it was time – the past and the future. 'Me used to have a lion with bells on, Dadda.' And she did. It is probably still under the sofa. One month it was lying, one month it was jokes. My favourite leap was nuance, the idea that 'Me supposed to have a chocolate egg' is a stronger formulation than 'Me want a chocolate egg' because it removes her desires from the equation. It makes the chocolate egg my problem. It makes it inevitable. (On my very favourite occasion, we passed an old blue gas tower, its sad gantries rusting and untended, on the edge of Brighton. 'Whaddat?' 'It's a gas tower.' 'Me supposed to have a gas tower one day.')

I sensed that a strange constellation was growing around Leon. Every day she would add – and I would add – to the nimbus of ideas and traits that I associate with her. That she is a performer. That she is a loner. That she is anything but a loner. This constellation of opinions about my daughter would grow so fast it soon felt like a little galaxy surrounding her.

And it was a danger. I knew this. I knew that this must be fought against. It is so hard to see our children the way they really are. This is the challenge, or a part of it. To see through our hopes for them, and our fears for them, to get at the simple truth of them from one day to the next, to understand and love the honest flux of them. And every day this gets more difficult.

One day this firmament around Leon will be fixed in place – an awful day when every fresh anecdote seems to start and end in the same way because it is getting at the same idea of her, because it has already come to its conclusions, because it is dealing with a caricature. This is the fate of all charts and all maps: one day exploration ends.

What I want, I decided one morning, waking up next to Leon and Sarah and glimpsing them, briefly, for one wonderful confused moment, as strangers, is to see these people as they really are, rather than to view them through all the lenses I impose on them. MS had made me aware of my perceptions.

Now, I thought, I must work out how to move beyond them. I must try to spot the things I am missing.

I was missing something important. Sarah and I both were.

In fact, we were missing something about perceptions. When Leon looks at books and toys, she holds them up very close. When she watches the TV, she stands right next to the screen as if receiving the unfolding narrative through the power of scent. All of this points to something so obvious, so utterly, inescapably obvious, that our own conclusions up until this time seem shameful. Oh, we had thought, Sarah and I, Leon is really one for detail, isn't she?

Well, she might be. But more pertinently, Leon is really one for not being able to see.

By late summer, we were back at the hospital. This time, though, there was a dark novelty: we were not there for me. The three of us were in the waiting room of the eye unit in Brighton, where we had been sent by a health visitor – her two-year check-up, and the last, somewhat implausibly, before she goes to school – who had noticed that Leon struggled to see pictures in books unless her nose was right up against the page.

Leon played on the floor of the waiting room where there were toys laid out. Sarah and I sat rigidly side by side: neither of us felt able to cope, but we were both just about holding it together by propping up the other one. This part of the hospital was old and due for redevelopment, and as a result there were marks on the floor by every door and wall that showed where the new doors, the new walls, were going to go. And they were close to the existing ones, always an inch or two apart, as if the building was having its own proprioceptive deficit attended to.

Except proprioception is my world, and this was all about Leon. I watched her play on the floor of the waiting room, and then I watched her, very intently, as she worked her way through a subjective eye test in the darkened office down the hallway. This initial eye test of hers: it was my first time really seeing Leon from the outside, seeing her as her own person, interacting with a grandmotherly optometrist she had just met, agreeing to try on a frame that allowed different lenses to be dropped in front of her eyes so the optometrist could see what happened to her pupils when she focused. Leon was calm and interested for the most part, sparking into happiness as toys were waved in front of her to draw her eye or test her ability to make identifications. She clapped each time she saw a mouse or a pony she recognized. Over time, she grew impatient, but only at the end did she stop cooperating entirely. I think the optometrist got everything except a good look at the back of her eyes.

Sarah had been making eye contact with me throughout all of this. We gripped hands, Leon on her lap, as the optometrist announced with great gentleness that our daughter was extremely myopic and would need glasses with quite a high prescription. 'They're going to start things off with half the strength she'll need,' she told us, but it was still high enough, we discovered later that afternoon, to make the salesperson in the optician's think we'd made a mistake when we told her the lenses we were after.

A few weeks later, after Leon was bribed into trying her new glasses on in town, she announced that she never wanted to take them off again. On the bus home, she stared out at the sea, at the sky, at the birds flying overhead and the buildings rushing past. The top deck, a seat to herself. 'Wow!' she said, again and again, pointing to a very normal part of the scenery and then another. 'Wow! . . . Wow!'

Over the following weeks, my fears for Leon, fears that have been floating around since I took her to see Brian, start to loosen their hold a little. Her world is not perfect, but it actually seems so much better than that. Her glasses reveal the character she has always possessed: she looks curious, witty, up for anything. Now, on the occasions in which she peers at the world very closely, we know that she truly is going for the detail.

'She got this from me,' I admit to Sarah, again and again, although it is already obvious, although we have been over it several times. Still I keep saying it, and I keep saying it because of the unspoken element. Maybe, I think – and I discover that I have never let this thought announce itself before – maybe poor eyesight will not be the only thing like this she gets from me.

I have an MRI in November, and then Christmas comes, the three of us at Sarah's parents' house by the coast, out on the very edge of England, wind roaring in the darkness each night as we play charades and bingo, and Leon fusses with the first toys she has ever asked for herself. I watch her playing in front of the three-bar fire in the living room and want, as I often have, to stop time and keep her here, in this moment. I recognize that once again, in this moment, everything is as I could ever want it to be.

January arrives. A new year, and milestones all around: Leon has her first haircut, bringing her back to the *Rosemary's Baby* look but with a young girl's face rather than a newborn's. She has her first mugging by seagull, a crucial Brighton rite, the bird swooping in on our way to the library one grey afternoon and snatching a twill of croissant from her fingers. 'He said thank you, Dadda,' she assured me afterwards. We get this from her all the time now: sentences, but also imagination, a new perspective on the world.

And then, one white-sky morning, I find myself wobbling on sea legs, stuck on the shifting deck of some ship while everyone around me seems to be on dry land. My brain feels like an apple bobbing on water. It is not unpleasant.

I walk up the hill to the hospital, swaying slightly as I go, to learn about the findings of November's MRI, which I have already almost forgotten about.

Another consultation room, another briefing as my ever-thickening medical folder is brought out. And as my sea legs have already confirmed, it turns out the drugs aren't working.

The latest scan has shown new lesions – one in the left cerebral peduncle and the other within the right frontal deep white matter within the superior frontal gyrus. Later, when I google these terms, I discover that the gyrus deals with self-awareness and laughter, among other things. It is handy that these go together. The peduncle, meanwhile, is a thing of horrible beauty: a weird bony plant that has bloomed in the midbrain and assists in fine motor skills, balance and proprioception. Best of all, if you search for *peduncle* online for any length of time, you will find med students preparing for anatomy exams laughing in shared disbelief at what an odd word it is.

Did I suspect the drugs weren't working? No. I didn't suspect it in the slightest, despite the mounting symptoms. And in fairness, the drugs *were* working. They worked beautifully, holding back the real terrors of MS and letting only the slightest of troubles through. The drugs were not at fault: I just had too much MS to go around.

Although there are ten drugs on the market now, most of them are less powerful than the pills I have been taking for a year, so they are of no use to me. This means that I am now left with one final choice. It's a choice between another drug that, once again, is very safe in terms of side effects but won't do much to hold the disease back, or a riskier drug, with a handful of potential side effects, that may not only halt my MS but perhaps reverse some of its damage.

I don't spend much time thinking about the safer drug. Instead, I listen as the riskier drug is explained to me. Lemtrada.

The nuclear option. An old chemotherapy drug that, if I choose it, will mean an end to pills I take each day, the *mennen* that Leon and I have a ritual about remembering every morning and evening. Instead, I'll be in hospital for five days on infusions, and then I'll spend a month in semi-isolation as my immune system rebuilds. My old pills dampen the inflammation caused by the lymphocytes, the roving attack dogs of the immune system, when they mistakenly lunge at the brain and dig into the myelin. These pills do this by suppressing the overall function of the immune system. Lemtrada, meanwhile, goes in and kills many of the lymphocytes outright, in the hope that, when new cells slowly remobilize, they will behave as they are meant to.

Sarah and I go through the drug company leaflets after Leon's in bed one night. While the spin is fiercely positive, the potential side effects are all listed.

The first potential side effect is fairly straightforward. After treatment with Lemtrada, some patients develop an over- or underactive thyroid. It's a common side effect, but it's also treatable.

The second, and less common, side effect is also treatable: Lemtrada can very occasionally cause a bleeding disorder in which the immune system destroys platelets that are required for blood clotting.

The third potential side effect is far less common, and far more dangerous. I can barely believe it when I read it in the leaflet.

Treatment with Lemtrada can, in extremely rare cases, lead to kidney disorders.

For a long time after Gene died, there was something I never entirely understood. I never entirely understood why he took that final risk – a last-chance transplant that, as I have always seen it, would either fix everything or end everything.

On a deeper level, what I have never understood, until I find myself looking through the Lemtrada booklet with Sarah, is that Gene wasn't ill – or rather, his identity was not entirely wrapped up in his illness. Some huge, vital part of Gene was still perfectly well, was still thinking about the future, was still planning, still dreaming, still wondering what to do with the rest of his life.

And this, I suspect, is the part that would make the treatment choice for him – the part that had a vivid, lively interest in the years ahead, in making the most of them. Everything about Gene, every memory, every anecdote, every instinct about him, led back to life.

That January when Leon and I went in search of Gene, I had felt that he had something to tell me, some advice to impart about how to survive in the strange world of the incurable. I could not hear his voice when I spoke with Brian and sifted through the pieces of him that survived in our minds. I could not hear it when I removed my glasses and searched the commuters of St Pancras for his ghost.

But I finally hear it as Sarah and I read about the side effects of Lemtrada. And I know I would have heard it now even if the third side effect had not involved kidney disorders. Because I finally understand.

'How do you feel?' asks Sarah that evening. I know she doesn't dread the decision, but rather the decision-making process, which, with me, is never pleasant.

'I feel good,' I say. And I do. And then I explain what I think we should do, and I ask her if she agrees.

I had time to wait now, a period of grace while schedules were arranged, while a bed was booked, while old medication was stopped and given a polite two months to flow out of me. This was a period in which I knew MS could return, unchecked, in any form, in which days began with no pills – although Leon still reminded me not to forget to take them – and in which I was waiting, I think, for a new lunging burst of sickness.

And one night in February MS lunged at me, out of the cloudless frosty skies of Blackfriars train station, the reflective black river merging with the towers on either bank to form a half-pipe of glittering lights. I was on my way to see friends from a game studio, an evening in a restaurant that floated by the dock in Greenwich. That was the plan. And then, as soon as I put my foot on the platform, stepping down from the train, countering the burst of vertigo I get from standing, a wind picked up and I found I had stepped into the thickest, heaviest fog I had ever encountered.

At the time, it seemed that MS had leaped out of the darkness, and while it had not made me blind, and had not taken me away from the world of things, it had broken that world with great suddenness into bright, sharp fragments that now lay all about. For a vertiginous second, this was no longer London, but a collection of lights and sounds and people pushing past in every direction.

Remember this, I urged myself as I swayed by the train, set rocking by a wave of awareness at my sheer sudden incapability to deal with the complexity around me. Remember how this feels.

The journey across London that I had planned and carried in my head like normal had disappeared; suddenly without it, I knew I had to get to a Tube map to rethink my next move. But when I found the map on a nearby wall, I laughed at the sight of it. Yellow and green and blue lines against a white backdrop. I knew that each circle these lines moved through was a place, but I did not know any more how to get to the circle, the place, I wanted to reach. I did not trust myself to enter this system of friendly geometry and jump from one line to another. I could not project myself into the map without effort, and I did not trust myself to apply that effort.

I must have tried a little bit. At some point, I found myself outside the station, walking a narrow corridor that led down to the sea. Not the sea: a river bank, a huge black river in front of me, the wind very cold, and everything around me, every surface, every edge, unnaturally sharp and bright. SEA CONTAINERS said the angled blue lights on one building. I nodded at it. SEA CONTAINERS. My phone buzzed. I looked down at the screen, itself clearer than I had ever seen it before, so clear I felt I could sense a greyness behind the light that was the image breaking down into pixels. I had been sent an email! I sensed it was important. The email was talking about balance transfer rates for February.

I knew it was February. I knew I was trying to get to a boat instead of the Tube. I breathed in and laughed again, delighted with the sudden emptiness, the silence, of my head, which seemed to allow the complex beauty of the world around me to present itself fully, in an unmediated form. I was not scared. I was calm. I was calm and cheered and rendered useless by everything I saw.

Remember this. I remembered I had come from Brighton, and I could probably go back there immediately. That seemed like a very good idea. I had a return ticket and I still knew – the memory was waiting for me – which platform I generally used to get home from Blackfriars.

I got on the right train and I picked up the paper on the table, folded over to the last page. A crossword. I knew about crosswords. I also knew I wasn't in the mood right now.

After an hour of empty-headed travel back to the coast, I sensed that my confusion had lifted. And I sensed, with a knotting in the stomach, that yet again some of that confusion was self-imposed. I had given up in the face of a difficult challenge, and maybe the challenge itself was, at least in part, yet another phantom.

No. This will not do, I thought. As I headed back to Brighton I texted Sarah, saying that I had to come home early but I was fine. Then, as I waited for a reply, I made a serious effort to go over what had happened. My confusion had felt so real, so complete, and yet did MS create confusions this deep and this all-encompassing, and did they emerge so suddenly?

And *MS confusion* suddenly seemed like a terribly broad term. Apart from my experience back with the IKEA bed, a lot of my MS fog so far had left me kind of dithery rather than completely emptied and bewildered. What I had just encountered was something far more comprehensive – something that I felt I would be reluctant to talk to a neurologist about, as it seemed tinged not just with MS, but with my hysterical, indulgent, useless reaction to it. And yet I did not feel hysterical any more, and had not felt so for weeks before this incident.

Might I be able to unpick this a little?

I went back to my arrival at Blackfriars. I have often drifted off on trains – which hardly requires the assistance of a neurological disease – and sometimes upon returning to the moment as a train arrives at a station and the doors hiss open, I have realized that my plans have floated off somewhere and cannot easily be regained. I remembered that from Blackfriars: the sense of suddenly being without a plan, and I remembered too that in MS it is acknowledged that the complex human stuff of making plans, of making decisions, can become trickier.

And I knew, as I had looked at the Tube map, that I probably could have pushed through the fog a little here – if only I had possessed the energy and the confidence to do so.

Lack of focus, muddled planning, and an absence of the requisite belief to pull it off. This suddenly sounded a lot like

MS to me. And yet this meant I was left with two conflicting experiences: I had worked myself back to an understanding that the
confusion I had felt wasn't actually very deep, and was mainly
about my ability to focus, to root myself back in a moment I
had briefly lost touch with. But I also had a vivid, panoramic
sense of what this was actually *like* to live through, the coherence of the world briefly fragmented, with few of the pieces
fitting together properly.

Maybe there was truth here. The truth that the mechanism
and the *effect* of the mechanism can be wildly different to comprehend. And maybe they should be. Unstitching a neurological
event can be a quiet business, calling for calm and clarity and
precision. But I do not live with precision, and I do not always
experience life with calm and with clarity.

I knew, whatever happened with Lemtrada, that I would
have to learn to live with this, with the knowledge that, on rare
occasions, there would be a gap between my attempts to understand something and my experience of it.

Maybe, over time, simply understanding that the gap was
there would help to close it.

The Viking Gene, the Equator and Vitamin D

The hunt for the possible causes of MS

One recent morning Leon woke me with the cheerful announcement that her fingers were tingling. Panic descended immediately. Thankfully, she followed this by explaining that she'd been playing a game for the last few minutes. She'd been testing how long she could sit on her hands before they started hurting.

As I calmed down, it dawned on me that I'd been so quick to assume the worst because this was one of those things I had avoided thinking about. Maybe now was a good time to confront it.

What are Leon's chances of inheriting MS from me? It is widely agreed that a person is at greater risk of developing MS if a family member has it. In the UK, roughly one person in six hundred has MS. The MS Trust cites a recent study that suggests that the lifetime risk for a person who has a parent with MS is one in sixty-seven. (This rises to one in thirty-seven if a brother or sister has MS, and one in five if an identical twin has the disease.) To add context, however, the Trust reminds us that one in twenty people over the age of sixty-five will develop dementia, and one in three of us will develop some form of cancer. There are over one hundred genes that appear linked to a heightened susceptibility to MS, but the fact remains that we are talking about susceptibility. Most people who develop MS do not have a family history of the disease, and while it has a complex set of genetic components, it is not classed as an inherited condition.

While I tend towards the belief that Leon's chances of getting MS are not catastrophically elevated by my own diagnosis, I appreciate that the whole subject is muddled. It is muddled by my worries about what my diagnosis means for her regardless of her own health, and it is muddled by the lingering uncertainty as to what actually causes MS in the first place.

There have been many hypotheses. Charcot, who acknowledged he did not know the cause of MS, spoke vaguely of problems of a 'moral order': grief, a loss of social standing and the attendant stresses. His notions do not strike me as particularly scientific. Others over the last century and a half have added their own theories: MS might be caused by overworking, by too much thinking, by certain sexual habits – they never said which ones – or by environmental toxins. Some theories have gained traction, such as the idea that trauma or prolonged stress serves as a trigger for a disease that is already present, but dormant.

The pronounced gender imbalance of MS was noticed early on – Charcot spotted that he had more female than male patients with MS in the nineteenth century, and today it is accepted that relapsing-remitting MS is at least two or three times more common among women, suggesting that hormones may play a role.

Equally, by the beginning of the twentieth century, many researchers were starting to look at the unusual geographical distribution of the condition. It is striking how much more common MS becomes the further you get from the equator. To take the most extreme example, across the Orkney Islands one out of every 170 women is affected by MS – an enormously high incidence.

The Orkney numbers are rising too. According to a *Guardian* article published in 2012, when Orkney and the Shetlands were surveyed in the mid 1980s they had a rate of 190 cases per 100,000 people. Now in Orkney alone, it's 402 per 100,000.

In recent years, the geographical shape of MS has put vitamin D firmly in the frame, since vitamin D is manufactured by the skin upon exposure to sunlight, and MS seems to thrive in colder, greyer environments. Many people diagnosed with MS, myself included, are found to have low levels of vitamin D when they present with initial symptoms.

Exposure to infection is also considered a potential causal factor, although the focus has moved away from the idea that MS is caused by a specific infection towards the notion that a range of infections might trigger a process that results in MS. Various viruses have been proposed as likely candidates over the last hundred years or more; the Epstein–Barr virus, which is extremely common, is now the subject of a lot of research in this respect.

Ultimately, the current thinking holds that MS is caused by a combination of factors, which would explain why its origins have been so hard to pin down. There are the genetic components to consider, along with the gender bias, along with vitamin D deficiency and exposure to an infection. And then there is a second tier of potential risk factors such as smoking and a form of vascular deformity that is sometimes present in people with MS.

Separating many of these elements remains enormously tricky, as the Orkney example illustrates. Some see the high incidence of MS in places like Orkney as an indicator that the disease is caused by what's often caricatured as a 'Viking gene', that it is, in part, the poisoned wake left by marauders from the north wherever they landed. Outside the Orkneys, other hot spots include Nova Scotia, Alberta and Aberdeen. East Kent, where I grew up, also has a relatively high number of cases compared to the average.

So is this proof of a strong genetic component – and a point of origin – or is it simply more proof of the role that vitamin D plays in the disease? Research published in 2016 found that MS symptoms appeared on average ten months earlier for every ten-degree increase in latitude. But there's an additional wrinkle: people born in an area with a higher than average risk of MS who then move to a part of the world with a lower risk assume the risk of their new area, but only if they have made the move before they reach the age of fifteen. (I was born in California, which is a low-risk area, but moved to Kent, a relatively high-risk area, before I started school.)

The search for a more complete understanding of the causes of MS is ongoing, as is the search for a potential cure. I am not expecting to see a cure or a solution to the riddle of why MS chooses one person and not another any time soon.

That said, I am eternally grateful that, when I look at Leon and fret that I may pass my illness on to her, I know a handful of things we can do right now to try to keep her safe. I can start by making sure she gets plenty of sunlight.

I still worry – I will always worry. But I do not feel entirely powerless.

8. Inside the Tent

Sunday

Sarah bought Leon a tent, a cheerful arrangement of thin tur-quoise fabric, dotted with strawberries and ice creams. Round and jaunty, it has a bendy frame inside that leaves the whole thing rigid but slightly tipsy, battered by strange winds. 'It's a circus tent,' Sarah explains to me, but Leon and I know that it's an explorer's tent. We set it up in her nursery where, surrounded by the toys she has only recently started to truly play with, it feels like a base camp: a first foothold on proper childhood.

Yesterday, I said goodbye to my endlessly indulgent employer and left the office to begin just over a month of sick leave – the hospital stay and then a long period of house rest while my immune system recovers. My last few features have been filed; I have achieved Mailbox Zero. This afternoon I am going into hospital for a week. For the first time in years I am not wearing a belt with my cord jeans, and I have no coins or keys in my pockets. 'It feels like I'm going to prison,' I tell Sarah as I put my things in a cupboard. 'You're allowed to wear a belt in hos-pital,' Sarah replies, but she knows that I'm not listening, that I have given into this fantasy of leaving worldly things, like belts and keys, behind.

Through sheer coincidence, I am starting a fresh notebook for my diary today. (My first note reads 'Saturday', which I immediately have to cross out because it is Sunday.) I am clearly flustered. I am about to get in the car with Sarah and Dad, but first I must say goodbye to Leon.

I find her in the tent, addressing a mixed group of dolls and teddy bears. Although it's early spring, it's hot out and the sun is shining. Everything inside the tent is tinted with a gentle turquoise light. Leon's happy to see me; she wants me to play with her and her odd friends. She is busy assigning roles by the time she notices that I'm crying. When she sees this, she doesn't start to cry herself. She withdraws, leaning back into her toys and refusing to meet my gaze. This is her latest means of reacting to a world that is not behaving: she will not engage. I back away, and minutes later I clumsily kiss her ear as she is carried past me, head down, to her grandparents' car. She is going for a trip to the park.

On our way to the hospital, I use the last of my 3G signal to google a rash. Sarah and I have been over the dangers associated with this treatment a few times, but not as many times, she admits, as she has expected us to. A vanishingly small number of people, we have discovered, have deadly complications from the infusion itself. Then there's the thyroid disorder, the bleeding, the renal problems, each one more serious, and less likely, than the last. At the gentler end of the scale is a rash I have only just learned about. The rash is almost a certainty. It's the rash I'm looking up now, so that I'll recognize it and won't freak out when it finally appears.

The rash is the most common side effect of Lemtrada. Every online diary I have read so far has mentioned it. There's a 90 per cent chance of it showing up. On the second day, or the third, the body reacts to the treatment, and this reaction starts to stain the skin red, archipelagos flaring up on the chest and arms, spreading along invisible fault lines, islands growing into continents that linger angrily before retreating. A hidden world blooms briefly, and then fades. A cartographic rash is the medical term, as I remember it. Close enough, Sarah tells me in the car. It's actually called a geographic rash, the body's classic allergic response to an invader.

Whatever it's called, on the screen of my phone these things have a belligerent prettiness. Nameless lands, separated by vast alien seas. Continents spreading across limbs.

The itching drives you mad, apparently, but all of that is secondary to me. The body will become a map. This is something I have understood for some time: ageing, illness, injury, the landmarks of life are noted down. The body will become a map.

On a brief trip to the ward a few days ago, I clearly caught the place at a good moment: golden bloom through the open windows, a group of women cross-legged on their beds, chatting and reading magazines. Lots of sportswear, as if everyone were taking a moment out on their way to the gym. I am introduced to somebody: Justine is having her third dose of Lemtrada later in the day. No rash yet, but it's been an easy run so far. She seems cheery in a way that makes me suspect she is always cheery. Everyone around her seems very content. People in the ward chat about the early spring, the animals in their garden that did not find the time to hibernate this winter. Illness seems a long way off. I walk away happy and realize that I have just broken a rule – a stupid rule that I have always known was stupid. I have properly met my first fellow MS patient. It was fine. It was helpful. I am incredibly grateful, in fact.

Today, however, the sun has already disappeared by the time I arrive. I worry the tone is set at the front door: as I buzz in, I am almost flattened by a huge man in mint hospital pyjamas, electrodes running along his bald head like braids. He is making a break for freedom, body frantic but an unengaged look in his eyes, as if the conscious part of him were sitting far back in its seat and waiting to see how this particular adventure transpires.

In the half-light of the ward itself I can see the various shapes of old grey figures, one leaning over a dinner tray, another propped in a chair. For now I ignore them all as I stow belongings and lie back on my bed, alternating between frowning at the open pages of an unread book and frowning at the soap dispenser that I am situated opposite. Reminders to wash your hands are tacked up everywhere. I read the signs in front of me over and over again. I will not look around.

Today, without the bloom and the golden light, without Justine and her gathered friends, this is very clearly a neurology ward. Fiercely blinkered, I am left to reflect, unkindly, on the fact that neurological disease inevitably does something to the voice. It gives each of the presences nearby a softened, gummy, early-morning voice. I think of splayed toothbrush heads, blunted pencils. Familiar stuff that has been worn down.

Sometime in the night they put a cannula in my arm, a needle with plastic mosquito wings, looking as if a small aircraft has crash-landed, nose first, in my skin. I stare at the valve of the cannula and feel its smooth edges. Sleepily, I watch a thread of bright red blood trapped within the line, rising and falling as I tilt my arm, like the core of an old thermometer. I have no idea how this small machine operates and yet that doesn't seem to bother me as it should. If I have a talent for illness, it is a talent for lying back stoically in the presence of great unquestioned assistance.

The cannula is surrounded by medical tape on which a nurse has neatly written the date. She flushes it through with saline solution, a chill that insinuates its way up the arm, briefly revealing secret causeways in a manner that MS has already prepared me for. 'Can you feel that?' she whispers, close in the darkness. 'In your throat? Some people can feel it at the back of the throat.'

I move my tongue around. Nothing. The last cannula I saw was mangled and broken-backed, put into Sarah halfway through Leon's high-speed labour, awaiting an epidural that never came, because there was no time for it. That cannula wobbled around and then fell out, and in the thrill of the moment we never really thought about what had happened to it. I forgot it entirely until I unwrapped it at home a week later, a Christmas ornament protected by one of my old shirts.

At night, the ward becomes frightening. A neurological ward with neurological shadows, grey and coughing in the darkness. Nothing good will come of this, I think, as I go to sleep. I actually see that sentence in my head, made visible out of sheer bitterness. I am a grumpy character in a comic strip.

I had hopes for this visit that went beyond MS therapies. Now I cannot put these hopes into words. Instead I think: Tomorrow, if I am well enough, I will be poisoned. And I will learn nothing.

Monday

I awake in the morning and find that fear has retreated. Is this resignation? Now I just want to get through the week.

I withdraw, as I have always known I would, into cold politeness. I am cheerful and brisk as blood pressure and pulse are measured, as I receive a Morse code transmission of pills, this dash for the stomach lining, this dot for anti-spasticity. Around ten, a pump is wheeled up to me, a wedge of scuffed grey plastic on a metal stand, and a clear drip is attached to the cannula in my wrist: antihistamines, which make me wonderfully drowsy and woozy. I stare at my fingers as the next drip is attached. This one has steroids that I'm warned will fill my mouth with the taste of metal. They do. It's always a relief when a hospital prediction comes true.

Finally, the chemotherapy itself is delivered. It is photosensitive, so it has to hide within a sinister black bag. There's an aspect of crow as it finds its perch on top of the pump. It is a charismatic presence.

I watch the fluid dripping slowly through its pipework towards me. I tell myself I should be alert for any change in how I am feeling, but although it's only eleven in the morning I've had a full day of chemicals by this point, and I am suddenly so incredibly tired.

I awake briefly to see a nurse squeezing the bag to force the last drops through. I awake again to see Sarah sitting next to me.

A nurse slides into view. 'Yes,' she nods, unhooking the bag. 'This is done.'

Tuesday

Something has changed.

I awake on the second day of treatment to find that this ward has its magical hour: five to six, when the light stains the ceilings a watery silver and the patients around me are briefly silent in sleep.

But the silence goes deeper. I have been awakened by my hands. This should be another dull certainty with MS, which gives me the first minute or so of every morning to prise my fingers out of clenched fists, to shake the arms and unpeel what feel like radioactive oven gloves — crackling with static that burns the fingers and advances all the way up the forearms.

But today? Nothing. I awake and my hands are lying flat by my sides. More: they are entirely quiet. No static. No tingling.

I wait, almost listening for the jabs and sparkles which I know must be coming. Nothing. I rub my fingers together and for the first time in a little over two years they feel cool and precise. The space they seem to occupy in my brain matches the space they occupy in the real world. I swear I can almost feel the whorls and counter-eddies, the vinyl grooves of my finger-prints, moving over one another.

I prop myself up on my elbows and sound out my other symptoms. Nothing there either. No hug gripping me in the ribs. No apple-bobbing as I move my head around only to feel my brain following it seconds later, turning sluggishly through water. But sometimes, I tell myself, this is the case anyway. Sometimes MS needs a while to get itself running properly at the start of a new day. *Sometimes* it even takes the morning off.

But never like this. The tingling fingers are my most constant reminder that I am different these days. They are never silent. They have not been silent for two years! Yet now they are.

I close my eyes and talk to myself, just under my breath. This is good news, I allow, but I am not going to run away with it. It is too soon for a reaction, for starters. It is psychosomatic, surely. Or it is the steroids. Of course it's the steroids. Still, I will give myself this moment in which the world has seemed to tilt and level out. I will allow myself this idea: not that the treatment will work, because who can afford a thought like that? I will allow myself this idea that I may survive the treatment itself.

As I rub my new fingers together I close my eyes and let the hospital build itself around me in my imagination, glossy and bright, first flockings of day nurses and porters in the squeaking halls. I am trying to get used to being a part of this particular world. It no longer seems impossible that I am here, that any of this is happening.

A nurse appears for morning observations. I ask her name: Annie, a towering cockney with a bob. I ask about a shower, and she says, in her sing-song voice, 'Let me just take care of this baby.' Not the pills, which are already swallowed: the baby is the cannula on my arm. She finds a bag to protect it from the water, and then, with wonderful unnecessary care, she tapes the bag tightly in place. 'I always fold the tape over,' she tells me with pride. I understand. It's so that I will have an easy tab to grasp when I remove it afterwards. Such a beautiful piece of work, I almost feel bad taking it off when I have showered. But not as bad as I feel in the bathroom when I realize the only way to bathe with a cannula in your wrist, bag or no bag, is to perform a prolonged Hitler salute.

I am still not ready to contemplate the crow. Instead, over the course of today's infusion, I try to turn this room of old men into people. The man in the far corner is Douglas, and he is not actually as old as I had first assumed. Disease has spun the dial on his ageing, it has made his handsome face drawn, and it has turned down the volume on his voice, with which he politely asks to be moved in and out of his chair as the sunlight advances across the ceiling, as the ward warms up.

Next to me is Phil, a tiny man, but a huge presence. His wild white beard and his curly hair both bounce as he moves his head, and seem to suggest an innate jolliness, but I know by now that he seethes all night, muttering endlessly as he tries to get comfortable, an angry Santa. Upon waking, though, he is full of confused life. He feels it his duty to entertain everyone, flinging jokes and remarks as the nurses come and go, attending to my infusion pump.

Opposite me and over by the open window is Edward, rangy and delicate. If Douglas is muted and Phil is sometimes mildly confused, Edward is present only in body. I assume stroke, until I overhear from the nurses that strokes were moved to County a decade back. We are something of a backwater here. Edward is in his sixties, I think, but only his early sixties, an aristocratic Indian man with glinting white hair. He seems completely empty at first, but the shell of past behaviour remains and becomes visible over time: a donnish gentleness, elegant posture, long fingers holding the *Telegraph* as he squints at the cricket scores. He is full of agitation, always trying to rise, trying to sit up and push out of his chair and race off deeper into the ward.

Out of the four, I am the only 'independent'. I am the only one who is allowed to get around on my own. As the steroids continue to rid me of any symptoms of MS, I start to feel lucky. Lucky in my youth, a cheery aberration on this ward. I struggle, really, to understand the pitying way that the others sometimes look at me. I wonder if the nurses think of me as MS, the way other nurses once thought of Sarah as polycystic ovaries. I remember that medical people do this, they lapse into this kind of protective shorthand.

The tingling in my left hand resurfaces quietly while Sarah is visiting in the afternoon. It is almost a relief: I can take good news, as long as it isn't suspiciously good. While I talk to Sarah about cheery nothings, I watch Edward across the room, and I worry about my dad bumbling around in here, an extrovert let loose in a ward where introversion has been imposed. Trying to start a conversation with Phil would be dangerous enough – and he is probably the best option.

An early ritual emerges. Every evening, once she has had time to return home, I send Sarah and Leon a text to say goodnight. Often it doesn't go through – we are in the basement, after all, although everyone still speaks of going 'up' to the ward, since hospitals mock and jumble physical space like nowhere else. I quite like it when the text doesn't make it, to be honest. The sense of separation lends a sweet pang to thoughts of Sarah, and thoughts of Leon, who is going to sleep many miles away. I can see her so clearly in her absence, sleeping, as ever, with a fat hand tucked politely under her chin.

Remember this. Remember that life is moments, that MS is a disease of the moments, and it says, in its swiping carelessness, that the moments matter. The silver moment on the ward where I awoke to silent fingers. The moment yesterday – almost forgotten – when a nurse woke me to say that Christ is her saviour and that my name makes her happy and will continue to even if I don't believe in him. Further back: the moment in the tent under turquoise light. Much further back: the moment when Leon first took my head in her hands and pulled me in for a kiss that she didn't yet know how to deliver, and she just hovered there, her mouth forming a smile, her breath on my cheek.

Wednesday

I get excited when a visiting neurologist asks Edward to read aloud from one of the books that line his window ledge, occasionally tumbling out into a stretch of garden when a nurse bustles past with an obs machine, which monitors vital signs. It feels like the whole room leans forward to listen. I instinctively think: Wordsworth! And then: Matthew Arnold? It would be hard to handle Arnold in here, the cauterizing shock of his bluntness, that brutal clarity of thought silencing the warm, muttering baseline of a place like this. T. S. Eliot would be too perfect, of course, but in the end I hear nothing much anyway. Edward's mumbling becomes a little more organized, falling into the sad rhythms of scanned text. This is the most basic act of reading: he can only glance off the words. Nobody connects. The neurologist nods and notes and moves on.

And I am left thinking – a kind of thinking, smug and speculative, that I recently suspected was gone for good. I think: Eliot really is perfect for hospitals, isn't he? And not just because of his etherized patients, his heavy limbs on heavy tables. He has that pacing rhythm that is perfect for the steady drift of time on a ward. His slow-tumbling associations are ideal for the sad thermals that thought must ride in the neurology ward in particular.

Then there's this:

> Who is the third who walks always beside you?
> When I count, there are only you and I together
> But when I look ahead up the white road
> There is always another one walking beside you . . .

I have never felt the need to understand *The Waste Land*, but years ago I knew the urge to understand this section. It led me to something called the Third Man Factor, which holds that an unseen presence is sometimes sensed in times of high adventure and extreme danger. Shackleton felt it on the glaciers of South Georgia, heading deeper into the ice. I do not believe it is a religious phenomenon. It is a regular feature among godless thrills, mountaineering stories, among any stories of survival.

And it fits so beautifully with neurology, with the quirks and feints and twists of proprioception. It fits here too, with the pump and the black crow of the Lemtrada bag tricking me into the idea of a presence lurking between Phil and me.

I think of a woman I once saw leaving the neurology department when I arrived early for an appointment. The first person I ever suspected was a fellow MS patient. I call her the Bird Lady, because of the same staggering walk on long legs, a taut, ruined grace to her. Days later I saw her again in town. I was rushing to work, and she was standing in a doorway, cane tucked under her arm and a camera raised to her face, snapping a picture of something that, passing the same spot again on my way home, I could not make out. Despite my cowardice regarding other people with MS, I was filled upon seeing her with a desire to make contact, a desire to thank her. To say to her that if she could keep going, if she could retain an interest in the world, so could I. I wonder now: has the Bird Lady had the chance to sit beneath this crow?

None of this is what I expected. I went into this expecting a communion with the worst of the disease. Well, a persistent drugged nausea, at least, or the blinding winces of MS headaches, lighting up the skull like a shower of meteors haphazardly streaking the night sky. Instead, it's been the opposite. The steroids have brought me back to my old life of oblivious healthiness, returned me to a place where the connections between things are easy to find, so taut and singing that they seem almost visible. I sense my own idiotic privilege in a place like this: how easy it is to be a good patient when you are already feeling well.

I sense, more, that truly I have yet to know what it is to not feel well. The jaunty obs machine is wheeled around every thirty minutes as the days begin to blur, and the fourth day – the third day of treatment? – starts to unseparate from the fifth, perhaps. This machine, blue and riding on many wheels, is the happiest machine in the world. It announces itself with the opening notes of *The Magic Roundabout* when it is switched on. It gives a brief sailor's hornpipe when it's done. And once the cuff and the finger clip have been removed, the news, for me, is always good. Blood sugar a bit high, but that just means the steroids are working. Heart rate and blood pressure remain textbook. Whatever happens, they never stop being textbook, even for an instant. A doctor, scanning my notes in a sudden midnight visit, seems almost angry at the consistency of it. He is suspicious, and so am I. I have come to hospital only to discover how obnoxiously healthy I almost am.

I am alone in that, in this ward, however. Douglas moves past, head bowed, pushed by nurses who clearly love him for his gentleness, the hint of humour he brings to his tiny shards of conversation. And Edward? I am becoming shamefully fascinated by Edward.

Edward's anxious restlessness takes a predictable form. He is stirred from bed not randomly, but in response to specific stimuli: ringing telephones, the bleeping of unanswered alarms, of which there are many in a hospital ward. When the electricians were in to fix a light, Phil asked them to leave because they were annoying him. Edward, meanwhile, staggered from his chair and tried to help them with the wiring. There was work to be done, and he was certain he should be at the centre of it. His battered mind has returned him to early middle age. Before disease. Before doubt. His illness seems to have picked a spot in the past when he was mobile and vivid and important, and now it is enforcing a cruel parody of all that.

Edward's illness seems particularly vicious. Each day it becomes clearer that it is offering an inversion of him, of his tendency to lead, of what I presume was once his extrovert nature. In health, he may have been a bit like my dad, but more rarefied, a touch dreamier. I still see his youthful energy in his desire to respond to every trill, to involve himself and to oversee every hubbub on the ward. I underestimated him, I think, until I see him one afternoon on the Zimmer frame, a pawn in a failed plot to use up some of that useless energy of his. On the frame, he is suddenly so fast, so astonishingly fast. Nurses need to slow him down, trailing after him as he races, head up, on some urgent, if indistinct, mission. He is dragging the frame one-handed behind him, but there is no mission. There is no destination.

Too much energy, and hence anxiety, as he feels there are things he should be doing, even when there are not. In life, he has looked after himself, which is probably a mistake. His body is ready for anything, but his mind has nothing to give it for the time being. 'There is nothing for you to do,' says the doctor. It is meant to calm him.

Phil is driven by old programming too, I suspect. He tends to misbehave when nurses and doctors are present, almost out of a sense that it is expected of him. He is playing himself, working his way deeper into an old role with every joke. He is a little scary at times, but he can be very funny too. During my third infusion, he raises his bed to its highest point, using a switch that nobody else has managed to find. 'Where are you going?' laughs the ward sister as he judders upwards. He points at the ceiling. Higher. A stately height.

And me? I wonder if I am involuntarily broadcasting arrogance. Silent except when spoken to, at which point my politeness is still almost brutal – an industrial pleasantness that must fool nobody. When I ask questions I think they probably suggest a desire to cross over, to be more than just the patient I am. I am curious about medical things, but I suspect there is also a passive-aggressive element to my queries.

Maybe I am more like Phil than Edward. Phil's jokes and come-ons show a lingering desire for control. He finds it hard to be at the mercy of people. So he places himself, in a comical sense, in charge of them. There is an imperious element to his jokey persona, and even to his occasional confused non sequiturs, a sense that it is a privilege for us to hear him speak. I love that. I admire that in a place like this.

I even listen in occasionally. I discover that nobody knows what is actually wrong with him. There is talk of sending him home. Beneath his faux dissatisfaction with his surroundings, he does not want to go home at all. 'I have only been here for two beautiful weeks,' he says. He has been here for six.

Often I read. I have chosen carefully: books to deliver the sense of exploration I need when confined to this place. Jay Rayner eating his way around the world; a history of the search for exoplanets; *Skyfaring*, the memoir of an airline pilot. It infects everything again, reading, just like it did before I had MS. When I need the bathroom, I take my drug pump in with me, its alarm bleeping rhythmically because it has been unplugged. Exoplanets intrude: it is like taking *Sputnik* for a walk.

A nice thought. Not just *Sputnik*, the pioneer, circling the globe, childishly announcing nothing but its own sheer and bizarre presence. But also that my mind can still catch things and make connections, even inane connections like this. Reading is still worth the effort.

In some ways, I am worryingly well suited to the small thinking that hospital demands. The simple pleasure of finishing another chapter, of keeping my cannula dry and pondering the next obs result. Of remembering who has taken Edward where and what kind of hot drink Douglas prefers.

In other ways, however, an old way of thinking is returning, a roving, self-satisfied autopilot that moves from one topic to another and seeks to tie everything together. Ugly as it is, I worry I have missed it.

And even as books give me back my old world, I wonder about it. I was delighted upon meeting Sarah when I learned that she hated to read – although she has since developed a love for reading anything about boats. I have mindlessly read too much of my life away. It's that Marcel Proust line I think about the most these days. You can live your life or you can dream it, he says, and if you live your life you will also dream it. Yes, Marcel, but if you only dream your life will you miss the living of it? I need more experience of living. When I get out, I hope I will not avoid life as thoroughly, as expertly, as I have in the past.

Another day is done. I do not know which day, but I could work it out if I had a pencil. It seems a hospital is like an

aeroplane. That sense of being in a holding pattern, that sense
of cooped-upness, of being sealed off from a world that suddenly seems very far away, far below. Today I read in *Skyfaring*
about place lag, the sense that on planes we travel too far and
cover too much distance for the lizard brain to truly make any
order of it all. Hospitals have the back-to-front form of this.
You seem to travel so long and so far that you can't believe that
you have not moved in the slightest, that the only journeying
done has been internal.

Like an aircraft, there is a chance to reflect on what you have
left behind, who you have become. Having a chair next to the
bed reminds me of the Third Man Factor. I constantly feel that
there is someone sitting there with me. They are pleasant but
watchful. Is this proprioception, or is this fatherhood? When I
lean back in bed at night and turn to the chair, I suddenly imagine Leon, grown-up, sitting quietly, *watchfully*. History in
that posture. Years of talking to a father as he lies in bed.

Thursday

Lemtrada is a clock. Each droplet is a unit of time, suspended
and then released by the hidden machinery of the pump. Drip.
Drip. Drip. I had a slight adventure this morning, or rather
Lemtrada did, when a new sister tried to plug in the latest
batch, hidden under its black hood, and the crow started to
leak. The liquid looked slightly thicker than water, and somehow brighter, as if lit from within. 'That was *very* bad,' said the
sister as she rushed to wash her hands, but it was only five mil
or so. Doctors were called, and doctors were unbothered. Five
mil is neither here nor there. I almost expected scorch marks
where it had hit the floor. Nothing!

Even in the midst of all this, it did not feel like real drama. The ward retained its measured pulse. Over by the window, Edward mutters, eyes closed. 'Gentlemen,' he says. 'Gentleman.' A cough. 'Fair enough. Fair enough.'

Day four of treatment? Today the rash will appear, I am told. Around lunchtime, maybe. The land will come up from the sea on my shoulders first, tiny islands, little lumps of angry red earth. Over time they will spread. They will join together. The full coastline will be revealed. I tell myself that I will understand something at this point, that a coherent way of seeing things is connected to that rising landscape.

Instead, departures. Rumours turn to news. Someone has died. I suspect it is the man in the single room across the hall, a shadowy presence, revered by us in some powerful way because of the depths of his illness. Not that we had a chart to go by – just the fact that he had the single room, which seemed significant. He rallied before he went, the nurses say. They often do, the nurses say, watching us, despite themselves, for signs of unwelcome energy.

Death is treated very beautifully here. Death matters. Voices dip. The shock is real. And the nurses respond with stories. Cath, a health-care assistant, remembers the minute her mum died – 3.03. She was knitting booties for Cath's unborn baby. Her mum was fifty-four. Now Cath is fifty-four.

And Phil goes home today. I will miss him, despite his occasional scariness. He fought the ward, which feels worthwhile, even if the ward itself does not deserve fighting. Besides, Phil has been a chance – there are so many of these – to see the wonder of the NHS in action. Everybody who has passed by, health-care assistants through to doctors, has offered to fix Phil's phone case, which he sat on a few days back in a fit, but only of pique. Everyone believes they can fix his phone case, even though Phil's own attempt to fix it has already rendered it permanently unfixable. He fought his own belongings as well as the ward.

Phil is setting off for the ceiling again, prior to going home. 'How long have I been here?' he asks. Today he thinks he has been here a week. His children are packing his things. His children are wonderful, small like Phil and blindingly fast and coordinated in their movements. Everything they do is done with great delicacy.

I hope Phil will be okay. Beyond his children, he also has the classic Brighton Jazz Friend helping out — I think you are assigned one once you hit fifty. Specs, sideburns, pork-pie hat and short-sleeve shirt, regardless of the season. A barrel-shaped man born to tap a hand on the steering wheel and mutter, wryly, about craft beer.

Edward surveys the hubbub of Phil's departure quietly, but a complex feedback loop kicks in once Phil is gone. I'm not sure how complex it truly is, to be honest, but it's certainly stressful. My pump runs down every now and then, and starts pinging to alert a nurse. The pinging sets Edward off: he struggles from bed to sort it out for me. I have to sit up to try to steady him, untangling myself from my various tubes as I go – and in steadying Edward from across the room, I only ever seem to beckon him over with increased urgency. He smiles to tell me everything is okay. He is coming to help! I grimace, because he is going to fall and it is my fault. The nurse comes in, and then it is a decision about whether to sit Edward down first or silence my pump.

No fat on Edward, and not in a bad way. He looks so healthy. Still ready for anything. After a week in hospital I can't help but see him in biological terms as he pads towards me. What a metabolism. A machine that takes care of itself too well.

Phil has become Harold, a new arrival on the ward. Minutes after they turn up, Harold and his wife are in the tent – the tent that is formed by the curtains around the bed being pulled, the tent that only appears when the doctor is visiting and people are learning difficult things.

After a short while, the doctor disappears, and Harold starts to set Edward off. Neurology has rendered Edward a programmatic element in some kind of simulation. He responds predictably to inputs, and now there are new inputs. When Harold rolls over and his bed squeaks, Edward rises to help him. And then Harold tries to get him to calm down, which only makes Edward more eager to help, which only makes Harold's bed squeak all the louder.

My own doctors arrive. Dr Koenig, my MS specialist, and Dr Quill, who I have not seen for a year, and who has not changed a bit. I find myself smoothing down the bed when Quill appears, organizing my books into a pile to show him how neat and tidy I am. My heart lifts to see him, and then falls a bit when he says, 'Because of this, the only downside is I probably won't see you very much any more.' He is being positive. Is he being too positive? I am not thinking about outcomes. I am not even ready to think about endings.

I nod to Dr Koenig as she leaves, and I think again of what she said when we first met: 'You will never be alone in this.'

You will never be alone in this. When I read in the afternoons, Leon is present as my bookmark. I prop her up in the last pages, so I am always reading towards her, as she glowers at me from a lovely, out-of-focus photo.

In truth, she is always present anyway. A change has occurred over the last few months, and only now am I fully aware of it.

When Leon was born, Sarah and I stared at her face for hours on end, rocking her to sleep, watching her wake, checking her for signs of tiredness or hunger or the first fluttering of social emotions. These were all excuses, though: we would have stared at her regardless, and as we stared we often ended up

seeing something familiar. We often ended up seeing the faces
of people we knew.

Leon, it was agreed, looked like me, and me alone. And there
is a reason for this, sadly: I gather that young babies look like
their father so their father doesn't run off immediately and start
another family. But the problem with this was that we also
agreed that Leon looked like Sarah, and Sarah alone. Except
when she looked like my dad, or my mum. Or Janey. Or Sarah's
mum. And maybe she didn't just *look* like these people?

For a while, in the absence of Leon's own personality, we
were projecting other people's personalities on to her. But this
slowly changed. For the last few months, I realize I have been
projecting her face on to other people.

A friend of Sarah has face blindness, which turns out to be
a neurological problem, prosopagnosia. She cannot identify
people she knows from their features; it is all just a jumble of
fleshy type to her, like swearing as it is rendered in a comic
strip. (It is not uncommon, incidentally; Oliver Sacks had it.)
With Leon, I have had almost the opposite problem over the
last few months – I will start to see her in the faces of people I
pass on the street, or even on objects if the mood grabs me.
Every trip into town will yield a few pangs from the crowds,
and I still get a bit misty about Henry, the vacuum cleaner with
eyes and a nose and a mouth – because they are so obviously her
eyes, her nose and her mouth.

I should have been untangling what it is about these specific
people and objects that makes me think of Leon. It's a chance to
learn what I most strongly identify in her. But I am left, instead,
wading through the clogging depths of emotion I suddenly feel
for these strangers and trinkets, the sudden spike of longing to
be back with her.

It is all education, with Leon. I am learning about her now,
with no thoughts to the way that she is different from the rest

of us or similar to the rest of us. She is reaching out to me, crossing the linguistic gap with each new sentence that expresses an urge, a desire or, increasingly frequently, a viewpoint on the world. We will be reading a book about animals and see – this is in Richard Scarry – a pig family riding in a car made of corn, all while they are eating corn too. She will laugh so hard that I worry she needs resuscitating, and then she will look at me and frown. 'This is funny,' she says. 'We should laugh.'

We should laugh, Leon. Leon, who thinks cars made of corn are funny. Leon, who has such a weird 1970s taste in food, drawn to cocktail olives, to salmon – to vol-au-vents, no doubt, if I knew how to make the wretched things. Leon, whose memory is terrifying, who can floor me, upon putting on a shirt, with a list of the recent and not-so-recent occasions I wore that shirt and what we got up to. Leon, the only Donlan who has ever invented a dance, who invents dances, in fact, whenever a new song plays on the radio, standing, listening for a second, before translating the music into movement, rolling the arms as if winding a bobbin, making chattering mouths from her hands, bending at the knees and then jumping like a frog.

In the evening, which is cool, I sign a waiver and promise solemnly to the sister on the desk that I will not fall over, and I go upstairs in the freight elevator that takes me from the ward to the wider world of the hospital. I am wearing a dressing gown and pyjamas and the two-tone shoes I brought with me almost a week ago. I feel dapper and crazy, unready for human company. I am listing to the left madly, as I am not used to walking. I don't fall over, though, and when I reach a phone signal I can feel the cool air of the evening on my face for the first time in an age. I call Sarah to hear about Leon, but all I can do is talk: about the breeze, the listing, the promise I made not to fall over.

She asks about Edward. I tell her about Edward. And I think:

I would love to have met him. There should be more to this sentence, I am sure, but I cannot untangle it.

Friday

Muttering retreats. In the cool light that fills the ward very briefly every morning, I see Edward, already up, already resting. It is before six and the morning observations: just the two of us and the bustle of nurses outside.

I watch his face. It is a delicate and cleanly sculpted face. I gather he was once a scientist, but he has the face, as the cliché goes, of a poet, easy and almost regal, with that aristocratic poise that tilts breeding towards battiness.

Actually, I think that Edward looks more like a poet than most poets do. Frowning over his book. The work of words churning somewhere within him. He certainly looks more like a poet than T. S. Eliot, whose face and laminated side-parting put him firmly inside that bank he worked for. Edward looks like he might work inside the head of a dandelion somewhere, his fine white hair a grasping of loose filaments as he tilts back and forth through the clear summer air.

Tethered to alarms, always stuttering to rise, a body that wakes each day filled with hurry, with the urge to take over, to restore order. And maybe. And maybe there is some order for him to restore after all. Maybe he has a message that he can impart.

Edward, I suddenly understand in the fleeting peace of dawn, is the last of my guides. He has travelled more fully into the wilderness of neurology, of illness, than anyone else I have met – certainly far, far deeper than I have gone myself. He has seen things in there. And this week he has been telling me about it. Or rather, I have been listening, with an increasing sense that I have been tuning into a signal that, while not meant for me, still has a clear relevance to me.

I think he has explained everything.

In a hospital ward like this, you get a chance to see what remains once the hollowing has done its work. And it's the Pavlovian stuff that remains. The rituals that have become hardened, that have become the stuff of neurons themselves. To fire together is to wire together: behaviour eventually becomes matter. Edward's desire to take control, to make us safe. Phil's desire to keep everyone entertained. A lifetime of programming is building up. What will be left when the conscious engine starts to spin down? It makes me wonder: what is my programming? What will be left of me?

Why did my thoughts turn to exploration so instantly when I became sick? And how have my thoughts shifted as my illness has advanced? I reached for exploration at first because I thought this was about being lost. I was deep into proprioception with its tricks, its shifting of the world an inch to the left. I recast myself as an explorer as a way of orienting myself – performing in metaphor that which the brain could no longer do for me automatically and invisibly. The further I settled into the role, the more I understood that what I was starting to focus on was actually a means of cataloguing what I was losing. I mapped my life to fix in place what felt at times like a vanishing world.

With Edward leading the way, dragging me behind his Zimmer frame, scattering nurses as he tracks down every ringing phone, every trilling machine, every unmanned desk and flickering bulb, I see that the thing to focus on is not what you lose but what you will be left with when everything else is gone.

Ben, Gene, Quill, Jennifer. Sarah. Leon. I was never an explorer. Explorers set out on their own. I was always looking for a guide, someone to follow. And it seems that I have always been this way, that this is the core of me, the part that has never changed. The middle child in a family of five children, loving the sheer rabble of us because it meant I never had to decide on anything, never had to create anything from nothing, never had to be the first to make a mistake, never had to pick a direction and set out to face something unprecedented.

But this? This is unprecedented. MS is unprecedented. For me and for everyone who gets it. You have to become the only expert. You have to become the only one. In some crucial way, you have to be alone with this.

That will be the last piece to go, I realize. All that will remain when the rest of me is gone is my endless need for help, my desire to get someone else to do the difficult stuff for me, so I can watch, record, follow – and occasionally lose myself in indulgences.

And more: in my endless attempt to understand all this in the context of other people, have I sidelined the people who matter the most?

The rash never arrives while I am in hospital. In the confusion of neurological disease, you sometimes get to the clear truth. As catastrophe pares you back, it is revealing something even as it destroys what surrounds it. You see what is left of people when they lose almost everything. Ben had anger. Gene had stoicism and hope, a sheer love of life. Edward has an innate need to help. Phil, a laudable kind of individualism. I think I have a deep-rooted need to follow, to be led to safety, and I don't want that to be my legacy. I don't want Leon to have a father who is still looking around for his own father.

Is this a big thing or a little thing? An air bubble, this is a little thing. This is surely the littlest thing.

One moment of drama before I leave. On my last day on the ward, my pump starts to make a new kind of beeping noise.

Not a gentle nudging beep, like I have heard before. Something a little more shrill: an alarm. The line has been fouled up, plastic flex bent out of shape. Annie, who can make wrapping a cannula for the shower a thing of precision and beauty, bustles over and resets the machine and checks the flex. She announces there is an air bubble in the line. She moves forward down the flex towards the point where it joins my cannula at my left wrist. 'There,' she says, pointing to a little valve set just before the cannula. 'I'll get it out there.' And then she bustles off to finish changing someone's bed.

I am calm. An air bubble, after all, is just a little thing. Dad, who is sitting with me, starts to panic. At least, I feel like he might be panicking. Messed up on steroids and woozy with antihistamines, I cannot completely comprehend his mental state, but I get a glimpse of it in the way that Sarah, who is also with us, starts to distract him, asking him about his youth in California, and his aunt, a favourite of mine who lived to be one hundred and two, kept alive by the stock market, which she monitored from her bed.

Annie comes back with a syringe just as the bubble is reaching the little valve. She does something with the needle and the valve that I cannot make out. It looks a bit like knitting, like casting off. 'All done,' she says, and bustles away again. I understand the rhythm of the ward by now, and so I know that she will be going home in half an hour. What I do not understand in the moment is that she has saved me from something serious, possibly fatal, and that she has done this with such a sense of calm, such a quiet, almost off-hand kind of competence, that it will be very unlikely if she thinks about it this evening or ever again.

Like Phil, I realize I don't want to go home. As my final infusion ends, as the crow departs for the final time, I hear Trump intruding from a TV in the nurses' station. Minutes later, hobbling around the hospital shop, listing to the left, I will resist the urge to buy a paper. I don't want to engage with global politics, certainly, but it goes deeper. I also don't want to engage with human currency, with pennies and debit cards and bank balances.

It is a struggle for me to say goodbye, but the nurses are used to it. They understand what they foster in their patients, and why it is so hard to put it into words. The car journey, the return home, and then Leon is where I expect to find her, in the explorer's tent, under turquoise light, and more beautiful and bright than ever. I have so much to tell her about where I've been. But it will be an age until she understands, so for now I hold her and she grins into my shirt and clings on tightly.

The Art of Diagnosis

I wonder sometimes what the last few years of my life have really been about. Have they been about multiple sclerosis itself, or about the paranoia and confusion that follow in its wake? Have they been about parenthood? Have they been, and this is a gloomy thought, about the slow, steady turn towards middle age?

Ultimately, I think a lot of time has been spent dealing with the idea of diagnosis: with the realization that a diagnosis was looming, and with my attempts to steady myself – and then re-steady myself – once it had arrived. MS is wrapped up in this, but so are my ghost symptoms, my many wrong turns. So too, and in a much happier way, is parenthood: someone was missing, and she is now here.

MS has a difficult relationship with diagnosis. Historically, its riot of symptoms has been hard for doctors to make sense of, particularly in the days before MRIs, and it is also not well understood by patients, many of whom will have little initial comprehension of the disease they are being told that they have.

And the moment at which diagnosis is delivered has sometimes been problematic too. One of the worst diagnosis experiences I have ever heard about I found as a footnote in T. Jock Murray's book *Multiple Sclerosis: The History of a Disease*. A female patient being diagnosed by Dr Samuel Alexander Kinnier Wilson in 1922 could still recall, many decades later, exactly what he had said to her. And he had said this: 'It's DS. Tough luck, old girl. You'll be in a wheelchair in four years. That will be five guineas.' (DS refers to disseminated sclerosis, an earlier name for MS.)

I say that this is only one of the worst diagnosis experiences I have come across, because for years with cases of MS it was often thought unwise to inform the patient of their diagnosis in the first place. Sometimes the doctor would tell a relative instead. Sometimes nobody at all would be told. I appreciate that MS is a disease that has had no viable treatments up until the last few decades, but it is hard to see the purpose in this dishonesty. It is also tempting to see institutionalized sexism at work, since the majority of MS patients are women.

I have become fascinated by the art of delivering a diagnosis. Over the last few years I have benefited from a diagnosis that was delivered to me with clarity, kindness and just the right degree of optimism. Dr Quill made certain that I understood the seriousness of what he was telling me, but he also ensured that I left with a sense that my life would continue, and that there were things that could be done and people who would care for me. At the many moments since my diagnosis in which I have lost my way, it is not because of the manner in which I was initially informed of my disease.

Dr Omar is an acquaintance of mine, a young physician who is planning to specialize in emergency medicine, and who regularly works shifts in A & E departments. As a result of this, he gives multiple diagnoses every day, and has a lot to say about the best means of delivering vital information to a patient.

'I do think that the packaging of a diagnosis, the words used to convey it, are as important to the lived experience of an illness as the concepts of a diagnosis,' he explained to me recently.

I asked Dr Omar how much he had been formally taught about this aspect of his job.

'At medical school we are taught about communication skills and things like "breaking bad news",' he said. 'So there is a general awareness of the importance of the mode of communication and not just the content. And medicine in the modern era of medico-legal paranoia and defensiveness means that you frequently see courses advertised for communication skills and so forth even aimed at senior doctors, not just junior ones. That said, there is a huge spectrum in skill that you witness in your day-to-day job.'

One thing Dr Omar told me about diagnosis has really stayed with me. He told me that with disease it is often a patient's 'story' that is truly broken. 'That phrase is not my own,' he admitted, 'but it means that it's their own conception of their life trajectory which has suddenly changed and been compromised as much as their physical function.'

This is yet another thing doctors have to take into account? I asked.

Dr Omar nodded. 'And I think it's important to be sensitive to this, to the football enthusiast whose broken ankle also breaks their pastime, their release and their fix of community, say. If done well, a diagnosis can be packaged with its implications and its impact on their life. Even better, it can be made a collaborative process, where you can work with a patient to identify how to tackle something that may impact them beyond just their body.'

Dr Omar was talking about an emerging branch of medicine called narrative medicine, an interdisciplinary

field that sees the way a patient's story unfolds as a
potential tool that may play a role in the process of
healing, if handled correctly, and may also encourage
self-reflection in the physician.

Narrative medicine appeared in the 1980s as a response
to an impersonal form of medicine that fails to take into
account the psychological issues that weigh on both
patient and doctor. It is not surprising that it emerged
during the period in which Oliver Sacks was writing his
case studies, which hum with compassion and curiosity.

'Clinical medicine is not biomedicine or physiology,'
Dr Omar argued, clearly falling into step with a favourite
subject. 'It is science as expressed through people, in
their symptoms and signs and their language . . . In the
diagnostic setting doctors are basically eliciting patients'
mixed-media stories, teasing them out and later recount-
ing them in a stereotypical, understood code.'

I suggested this sounded pretty complicated, but Dr
Omar said it felt like a natural process. 'When doctors
are talking to patients they are speaking in story,' he said.
'When doctors discuss patients with their colleagues they
speak in stories; when they document a patient's sprawl-
ing account in the ordered, mannered form expected of
clinical documentation they are just translating a story
into another type, one that makes things neat and treatable. Stories are what doctors deal in, and are the
construct by which doctors know illnesses. This is an
unspoken, often unseen aspect of clinical medicine, that
single words or turns of phrase can be pivots around
which a whole diagnosis and a life can change.'

That insight could have come from Sacks himself, I
think, a man who understood that it is fairly easy for
disease to become a story in the first place, and who

knew that, if you are particularly unfortunate, disease can become the only story.

I have still not told Leon about my illness in a way that she can understand. She knows that I take pills every day – even now I take a few every morning and lunchtime for spasticity – and she knows that there is something wrong with my brain. But I am waiting for the right moment to explain everything, to 'speak in story' about my illness. And that means waiting for when she is ready to hear it, and when I am sure I know how to tell her.

9. The Explorers' Club

We took a trip recently, just Sarah and I. We set off in a little boat, chugging out towards the horizon to see the wind farm that has been slowly coming together at the limits of Brighton for the last few years.

This wind farm has bewitched Sarah from the start, its strange, spindly architecture calling to her ever since it began to rise out of the sea. People sometimes ask Sarah why she's become so obsessed with the boats that come and go in this plodding stretch of the English Channel, why she downloads apps that allow her to track nearby craft, why she collects books on maritime lore, on wrecks, and why she spends so much time on the bus staring out at the wind farm as it spreads across the horizon. She can never offer much of an answer, or rather, she knows that no single answer covers it all. Is it a reaction to suddenly being so close to the coast? A way of getting a breath of air, when all three of us are crammed into a tiny bungalow? Is it a bit of distance from all this talk of neurology, of treatment plans, of so much helpless fretting?

We have all succumbed to the wind farm a little. Across the last few seasons, it has tangled itself with our waking and sleeping hours. I report back on progress when I get the early bus to work on a Monday, and friends living further along the coast tell us of clear nights when they can hear the sounds of construction drifting over the surf. Even Leon has looked at the farm through the binoculars. She has looked at it for a few seconds anyway, before she is distracted by the clouds, by the birds, by her own thoughts.

It feels dangerous to get up close to something that is so perfect from a distance, gleaming metal poles arranged in neat lines, strung with improbable rigging and lit by the shimmering point at which the sea meets the sky. We head out with a local dive captain who has gambled on running a tour of the turbines.

It is eight nautical miles from land to the wind farm, and that is space enough to watch the sea move through many forms. As we leave the marina, Leon and her grandma waiting on the dock, the water's an oily mineral green, little white peaks bouncing away from the bow. Twenty minutes from land and thick cords of froth are tumbling and tangling in our wake as we pick up speed.

Sarah's giddy with happiness. Forty minutes out and we suddenly notice that for the last few miles we've been entirely alone, Brighton disappearing into the yellow bloom to the rear of us, while around us buoys are the only landmarks, bobbing frantically as they pull against submerged tethers. It does not take much to leave the world behind, and in its absence we grow quiet and introspective.

'I've been thinking about what happened,' says Sarah. She's almost shouting, but over the chug of the engines it still sounds like a whisper, warm and conspiratorial.

'It is an adventure story,' she says. 'But I'm not sure it's the adventure story you think it is. Is it Lewis and Clark? The Northwest Passage? Or is it *Don Quixote*?'

The minute she says this, it starts to make sense. 'Don Quixote, driven mad by his reading, by his dreams of the way things are meant to be,' she continues. 'With me as Sancho. Now and then.'

She laughs. 'A story of perceptions and misperceptions.'

She leans in close. 'And since we're all Don Quixote really, I guess that means you're still one of us.'

My dad told me once you should read *Don Quixote* three times in your life.

'So you're saying,' I say to Sarah after a lengthy silence, 'that you don't need to have a neurological disease to misunderstand your own life?'

'Yes.'

'But it helps?

'Absolutely.'

Another buoy bobs past. 'All this self-knowledge, and nobody had to die,' laughs Sarah. I think about this too. Nobody died. But something did. My complacency died, and I slowly realize I was better off without it. Maybe it was years of complacency that were now making me feel so anxious about everything. I don't miss that sense of my own invulnerability that I must have had before this began.

It's cold this far out from land, and a slight breeze is picking up by the time wind-farm platforms start to appear around us. They're beautiful and stark: cylinders painted a bright yellow, topped with gantries and cranes. These platforms are the little stubs we can see from the coast road, the bases for the turbines themselves. Out here, they already tower over us, but they're still only a fraction of their final height.

For the last few minutes we've been able to see a complex grey mass on the horizon, 'It's the *MPI Discovery*,' gasps Sarah, star-struck by her favourite vessel suddenly up close and looming. The *Discovery* grows bigger and bigger before us, losing none of its alien nature, its industrial surrealism, as we approach. It looks like a freighter, a mini tower block at one end attached to a red hull – but that hull itself has been lifted out of the water by those thick metal legs that reach down beneath the waves.

Soon we can see the sun reflecting from windows, thin lines of cabling stretching from cranes and pylons. At the stern is a

giant propeller, raised clear of the water and hanging in the
morning air. The *Discovery* seems weird and perfect resting
above us: an improbable tool for the construction of an improbable project. I tend to think of otherworldly things as being
insubstantial, ghostly and gossamer, but this vast ship, lifted
out of the sea and hanging on the horizon, is the most otherworldly thing I have ever seen.

On the way home, we sit towards the back of our boat. There
is a diving frame, made of some sort of scuffed silver metal,
standing over the stern, a strange doorway opening out on to
the ocean.

On a Saturday morning before I had gone to hospital for my
Lemtrada treatment, I had sat with Leon in a restaurant in
Brighton. The light was good and Leon was in a sweet
mood, swinging her legs beneath the table and delighted that
the days of highchairs were behind us. While we waited for
drinks, I pulled out my phone and took about thirty pictures of
my daughter, one after the other, for no good reason beyond
the fact that she was there and so was I, and the phone had bat-
tery life and a bit of storage. When I look at the pictures now,
what amazes me is the difference between each one. From
one picture to the next, her expression is always changing.
She's bored. She's delighted. She's hungry. She's considering a
complicated idea. She's spotted someone she thinks she knows.
She's pretending to be a pug. All this in the space of fifteen
seconds.

This is a glimpse of the speed of thought. Or, more specifically, it is a glimpse of thought as it exists during the early
starbursts of myelination, when it is rangy and overwhelming,
and when there is nothing between the rushing conception of
something new and the way it tugs at the facial muscles. As
with so many things about Leon, it delights and frightens me.

So much is happening to her every day, which means there is so much to be missed.

It's all a bit cruel: for the time I was apart from Leon in hospital, I think I became the parent I want to be. I slowed down, ignored the phone – it didn't work anyway – and I read books and allowed reading to carry me back into a world I had missed. I watched people, perhaps too much. I thought about people I knew and would like to see again.

I return home from hospital to the tentative pleasures of an early spring, and the geographic rash finally flares and then fades. Red islands, raised and felty, spreading around the chest and waist, forming archipelagos that seem to reach out from one wrist to the other. They burn, these fresh landscapes, but only softly. They warm me.

As the red marks recede, I realize that I don't want the virtues I fell into in hospital to fade as easily. The first morning back in my own bed, I instinctively reach for my phone upon waking. As my hand closes around it, I suddenly understand, with a faint nausea, that I don't want this. I don't want to start worrying about the games industry. I don't want to start fretting over social minutiae or poking around Amazon for books that will go straight on to the shelf because there is no time yet to look at them.

For the weeks leading up to my hospital trip, I was off my old medication, and off any medication at all, except some light things to deal with spasticity. I got a chance to see what MS might be like with nothing between me and it.

When I had last experienced it without drugs, it had still been a little thing. But now, without my pills to protect me, it was a big thing. It was like a great wall approaching, like the huge flat face of a bus rushing up and hiding everything on the other side of it. Full-blown MS, even at this early stage, can be an insistent and bullying disease. It wants all your attention.

And it will have all your attention. I couldn't focus. I could barely do my job or talk to my wife and daughter. I walked into things. (There is a joke about this: *A person with MS walked into a bar.* That's the entire joke.) I regularly forgot what I was doing while I was doing it. I couldn't sleep because of spasms in my legs and arms, and every trip into town required regular rest stops: you need vast reserves of small talk for that kind of walking. Why talk, though? All I could really engage with was this thing that was pushing up against me, this endless distraction.

Now at home, as the hospital drugs wear off, MS starts to intrude again, but it feels much gentler. For a few days, it is just familiar electrical sensations, a friendly tingling and glitching.

Four weeks of isolation follow my infusions. Four spring weeks in which I am unable to leave the house or see anyone apart from my immediate family – this amounts to Sarah and Leon, the only people I really want to see anyway. Our tiny bungalow on the outskirts of Brighton becomes a spaceship. The porch becomes an airlock where Janey drops off packages from work and the odd cake. I wave at her through the window as she backs out, wheeling her son in his pram. A developer sends me a massive card, signed by everyone on the team, and I find myself crying for an hour: they make a game that is concerned with pure freedom, in which you are a robot who is also, undeniably, a child, and you soar through the air and explore rocky islands that float in the sky. Freedom! I look out of the window and watch the wildflower garden on the green starting to come back to life after the winter. The grass grows glossy and pleasantly ragged. Soon the sparse and scattered trees will be rushing into pink blossom.

It is perhaps slight overkill to stay in the house, but I am anxious to do all I can to avoid infection. I have little immune system to speak of, so I have to wash my hands constantly. I manage to duck most problems. To avoid listeria, I need to ask myself before eating something: Do the French like this? Eggs, dairy, sauces, cold meat? If it's too French I have to skip it. A strange rule of thumb, but it seems to work.

For four weeks I get up late and stumble around a house filled with sunlight: light from all angles, a golden bloom erupting in every room. It seems crazy that I could ever have struggled with this place. It is beautiful, compact and strange, all those rooms coming off the centre, with views of the green offering cameos of crows and magpies and the very occasional pheasant, witlessly elegant and still. At night, fox cubs dance and spring in the garden while their mother patrols, head held high against the darkness. I sleep during much of the day, but I am often awake through these quiet hours, happily staring out of the window, even when there are no darting animals to draw my eye. Happy just staring into space, I am at my mindless best. I remember that I used to worry about middle age. I saw it as a dimming of curiosity. It now seems that I am just as curious as I ever was, in every sense of the word, sadly, but the things I am curious about have shifted, to birds and to foxes.

Over the course of this month indoors, my symptoms slowly return to something that approaches my pre-treatment levels. My left hand is lost to static once more, as I suspected it would be, and my spasticity is back. My eyesight had deteriorated over the last few years – I very much doubt this is MS, to be honest – and I have to buy a magnifying glass to read my phone, an affectation that is so perfectly suited to me that Sarah doesn't even notice it at first. It is like when I first told my friends I had MS, and that one day I might have to walk with a cane. One of them frowned and looked at me with his head tilted. 'Don't you walk with a cane already?'

The very worst of MS remains on the periphery, though. My word-finding problems are reduced, my occasional stumbling in sentences largely gone. Four weeks is a long time to sit and think about things, but I don't think about MS as much as I expected, and this feels like a victory. Also, my right hand has stayed entirely clear. It is still mine. I spend hours staring at my fingers and flexing them, as if doing one of those magic tricks where the knuckles become an endless staircase that a coin can tumble down for ever.

One night in early autumn I decide that it is not just our job to keep Leon safe. We must show her the world, if we are able to. I have been listening to an interview with the New York magazine food critic Adam Platt, and he has been talking about his childhood as the son of a diplomat, which meant he was constantly being sent to distant parts of the world to start over in new surroundings. The quickest way to understand a new place, he says, is through the food, and then he tells a story about being eleven or so and visiting a Vietnamese restaurant surrounded by rice paddies, where he would drink Coca-Cola from a thick glass bottle that he would then hold on to because outside there were people selling rockets that could be launched from the bottle high into the sky above the paddies.

'We need to take Leon somewhere,' I say to Sarah, as we are sitting on the sofa watching the green.

'Barcelona?' Sarah replies. There is no money for Barcelona, but for once that doesn't stop us. Maybe we are both a bit disinhibited these days.

We are in Barcelona in November for the American election, which feels like another diagnosis, just as Brexit did a few months before. On the day Trump wins, we go to the Museu Picasso, where there are a handful of rooms devoted to Picasso's struggles with *Las Meninas*, by Velázquez. The greatest of all paintings, bringing distant historical figures to life before you. Velázquez's vision is starkly, arrestingly domestic, if such a thing is possible: it always shocks me with its sense of bustling life interrupted. Picasso renders his version in blacks and whites and greys on one huge canvas that dominates the first chamber of this section of the gallery, and then he breaks the image down into sections and characters that line another few rooms.

It's systematic stuff: hard work, and you feel the effort. The Infanta becomes a ghost, and then a Tube map. The dog is replaced with a piano in one picture. The windows of the chambers at the Alcázar that Velázquez has shut are opened, hundreds of years later, and light bursts in. As I stand there with Leon squirming and bored in my arms, legs gripping my waist, I think: This work of Picasso's, it is glorious and slightly pitiful all at once. It is an attempt to understand something that cannot be truly understood. Today of all days this approach feels so valuable.

I must return to the world, I announce, and once Sarah has finished laughing at my loftiness, she agrees. I must return to caring about things properly. MS turns you inwards, I think, and I was pretty much turned inwards even before that. It is time for a change of focus.

And Leon is the perfect inspiration. She loves travelling, and she takes to everything with ease. One night we are up past ten, and she's eating pasta in an outdoor restaurant surrounded by lanes of hooting Spanish traffic. She is completely unflustered as she spears chunks of minced beef on a fork that seems huge in her hands. You'd think she had done this every day of her life.

She is changing. Her voice has picked up a lovely aristocratic croak – she sounds like Dorothy Parker, or a sarcastic frog from a fairy tale. And she is allowing, for the first time, doubts to enter into her world. On our last day in Barcelona she wants to play hide-and-seek in the apartment we're renting. She counts to ten in the living room, and in the second bedroom I duck behind a table. Her counting drags on longer than expected – she has forgotten nine again and wants to go back and get it all in the right order – and I find myself checking my phone. Looking up bus connections to the airport maybe, or a neurological curiosity I read about the night before. An aphasia, an alexia, an agraphia, a dysnomia. Neurology has all the best words.

I lift my head from my screen just in time to see Leon enter the room. She doesn't spot me, which means that for a second I get to observe her as she is without me, wide-eyed, totally free of guile, an eager, open face driven by curiosity. I am about to wave, but she ducks out of the room again to continue her hunt. I hear cushions shifting around, floorboards creaking, and then, a minute later, a quiet voice.

'Daddy, I don't want to play any more.'

In the seconds it takes me to get to the living room – and for Sarah to burst from the shower – Leon is sobbing madly, face down on a sofa.

'What's wrong?' we ask. 'What happened?'

'I thought you left me,' she heaves out once she can speak again.

Leon, we would never leave you. We would never leave you. In fact, it feels like I have only just started to really see you.

This story of mine. I knew this story, until I tried to write it down. Then I noticed it was not quite the story I had been telling myself it was.

I recently sat across the table from a neurologist – not one of my own neurologists – for an hour and a half and listed all the things I thought had happened over the last three years. All the glimpses of cognitive decline, all the unmade beds, the unopened doors, all the vanishing stutters, the thefts of words and the fogs descending at train stations. How much sounds real to you? I asked. How much sounds like MS? A lot of it, he said immediately. Maybe even almost all of it. But, he added, you will never get two neurologists to agree on anything, so set yourself some different parameters for the evaluation of your own experiences.

I don't know, the more I look back at it, whether my reaction to my diagnosis was appropriate. Whether it was useful, for myself or for the people around me. I wanted to see MS as an adventure, which sounds ridiculous now, but still. I wanted to see it as a chance to explore this new world I was suddenly lost in, a chance to find my own place within it. I set off to discover the truth. And then I lost my way. And then I made life difficult for everyone around me. Is that my story?

I am aware that not everyone reacts to MS quite so catastrophically. I suspect that the majority of people don't. At a blood test in the neurology department a few months back I was signing in at the front desk when an energetic man raced through the front doors, skipped the queue and disappeared inside. He was youthful and gloriously full of bounce; I assumed he was a physio. But he wasn't. I saw him minutes later, emerging from the MS infusion team's room with a cotton swab taped over his arm. He disappeared whistling and I felt shamed by his briskness, his chirpiness, by the small space that I decided MS must occupy in his life.

And it's not just MS. Here are two approaches to bad news that I like. Fergus Henderson is the chef behind St John, a restaurant that serves bone marrow on toast, Eccles cakes with Lancashire cheese, and a brain burger, if you ask for it, which he says tastes like a crispy cloud. Upon learning that he had early-onset Parkinson's, Henderson felt glum, he often admits in interviews. And then he had a nice lunch and he felt much better.

Or there's Wallich. In 'The Schreuderspitze', a short story by

Mark Helprin, Wallich is a photographer living in Munich at the start of the twentieth century. His wife and young son are killed in a car accident and, silenced by grief, Wallich leaves his business behind and flees to the Alps, choosing a village with a name so stupid that he knows his friends will be embarrassed to visit him there. One day, the idea arriving fully formed out of nowhere, he decides that he is going to climb a mountain, so he starts to prepare for this difficult task. He reads books on mountaineering. He trains himself. He makes some pieces of mountaineering gear from scratch and buys in the pitons and special ropes he will need at great expense.

And then, when his kit is all arranged and his preparations complete, he starts to dream. Over the course of three nights he dreams the entire ascent, the perils and the beauty of moving from rock to ice, of facing desperate challenges and relying on hard-won knowledge to overcome them. On reaching the summit, he suddenly understands that the mountain he's climbed is much taller than he initially thought it was; it is *so* much taller. The entire world is suddenly spread around him, glittering and bright. And when Wallich wakes after the dream of his ascent, he gathers his belongings, heads for the train station and returns to Munich. He understands, you might say, that he must return to the world.

It would be impossible, I think, not to identify with Wallich in this story. But maybe what I mean is that it would be impossible for *me* not to identify with Wallich. The first time I read 'The Schreuderspitze', long ago, back when I could still discuss it with Gene, and probably did, I thought: I would do that. I would do exactly what he did if something of that magnitude happened to me. And now, reading it again, I think: I may not have experienced something so boundlessly vast and terrible, but when experience came for me, I *did* do that.

Recasting myself as an explorer seems, in retrospect, like an indulgence. A way of misleading myself. But I never felt I was giving in to bullshit completely. At the start of this, I felt like I had a decision: I could retreat into my diagnosis or I could see it as a starting point, a chance for something positive. I decided I could be a victim or I could see the wide world of neurology as something vital and interesting and filled with hidden possibilities. That mindset allowed me to deal with something that was otherwise overwhelming – even if it opened the door to phantoms.

And all that worry about the ravages of the mind allowed me to look away from the potential ravages of the body. These are arriving with more force now: the pain and the stiffness of spasticity, the jabbing in the fingers and the palms. A hug that once popped up in the evenings, around six, and lingered for an hour, now wakes me in the morning and retreats only when I go to sleep at night. My left leg is sometimes rigid as I move, and so my neck often hurts because I stretch my head to the right in compensation. I walk funny some days, and I am handling it. We are handling it. Sarah talked to me about cruises last week. I have never wanted to go on a cruise – it strikes me as paying to spend a week in a multistorey car park that wobbles – and she has always wanted to. 'We'll have to go on them one day when you have mobility problems,' she said last week.

I laughed. 'Do you think I'm going to have mobility problems?'

'Of course,' she said. 'But I don't mind. I don't mind *because I've always wanted to go on a cruise.*'

It is now spring 2017. I have had MS for three years. How am I doing? I *tell* myself that I am doing well.

Talking to my dad recently, I said that I had discovered a great secret – one that I didn't really know what to do with. We were driving to a blood test, a monthly affair to monitor my ongoing reaction to Lemtrada. Although my dad lives hours away in Wiltshire, although he hates Brighton so very much, he insists on taking me to my appointments at a hospital that is only about forty minutes from my house. It is a ritual that I love: a chance to catch up on things, and perhaps a chance for Dad to monitor me for any signs of MS personality. Although I know that the clumsiness of his initial warning has become something of a wound to him, I, in turn, worry that he was more right at the time than he knew. I am grateful that we have such a close relationship that we can be so clumsy with each other.

'Where did you learn this secret?' Dad asked, taking his eyes off the road just long enough to miss our turn and trap us on a roundabout for a few hairy seconds.

'In hospital,' I said. 'It's not a discovery, I suppose. More of a realization. I've realized that it's the job of a parent, the final job, the secret job, to die for their children.'

Dad said nothing, but his relaxed positioning in his seat, one hand on the wheel, seemed to stiffen.

'Not die in the sense of rescue them from a fire or throw yourself in front of a tram for them,' I said. 'But you die, eventually, to show them that it is okay to die. It is the final thing you have to do.' I laughed, although none of this was particularly funny.

Dad thought about this as he drove. The road curved through trees, the petrol station that marks the perimeter of my hospital appeared, and I realized I did not want it to appear just yet. I wanted to keep this moment going a little longer.

'I guess,' Dad said, 'that I see parenting as dying well, but also living well.'

Now I said nothing.

'Not living gratuitously, or luxuriously,' Dad said. 'But

living in a way that gives your kids a template they can follow or ignore but hopefully not be too embarrassed by.

'That said,' he added, 'they'll be embarrassed anyway.'

We came to a stop. Dad leaned over and popped the door for me, and I nodded and went into the hospital. I was on autopilot now, stopping briefly to sanitize my hands by the front doors and then heading inside.

All this time, I thought to myself, this has been the real mission, hasn't it? To find a way to live well. I thought of Ben in Worcester with his kids and his family car. I thought of Brian and his ease with Leon. Find a way to live well. Gene found it. Have I?

And this: 'To show your children it is okay to die.' In the days after that conversation, this phrase among all others will not go away. It feels so true, so unarguably true, that I am certain it must have come from outside of me. It must have slipped in from a favourite book, a favourite writer – it sounds kind of like Martin Amis? Helen Macdonald? Michael Paterniti? – or maybe a song, a lyric I once heard and then forgot to forget.

I spend a weekend looking through bookcases for anything that could have birthed it, and scouring quote sites online. I cannot find it.

Or rather, I have not found this thought expressed in exactly these words. In different words, however, it is absolutely everywhere. I see it in a remembered line from Gene's humanist funeral on a rainy day in Golders Green, when we were all told, and we all believed, that there is no life without death. It is there in that line from Saul Bellow, so often quoted by Martin Amis, that says death is the dark backing a mirror needs if we are to see anything in it. It is there in the line from the Episcopalian funeral liturgy that reminds us that 'in the midst of life we are in death'.

This sentiment is all around us, and buried within it a secret instruction: to face death and acknowledge its power, and to acknowledge the equal power of life.

Every month, after Dad drops me off at the hospital, I arrive in the neurology wing where my brother was once treated. When I first entered this wing, when Ben was ill, it seemed vast and terrifying. I got lost on my way to the drinks machine, to the car park, to the ward, on my way back from getting lost in the first place.

Now, though, in 2017, coming here is something I almost look forward to. Early spring feels like summer down on the wards, bright light coming in through the windows and making the halls and visiting rooms seem airy. I know many of the people I pass well enough to nod to them. The news from my tests, so far, has been tentatively good, and I am prepared, I tell myself, for the news from a forthcoming MRI to be considerably less good.

One thing has been missing, though. I noticed recently that, as I walk these halls to and from my blood tests, I still tend to think that I am somehow singular. When I pass other patients, I sometimes wonder what it is they are here for, but I never ponder the chance that they might have MS. I have cut myself off from this thought since the very beginning, since I first met Jennifer. And over the last few years my fear of meeting someone with MS has changed into something far more ridiculous and self-involved: I have started to think that I am the only person around here who has MS.

The corridor where I sit and wait for my blood test is one of the special places of my new world. I am always on my own down here. Dad may drive me, but I make him wait upstairs, and I would never bring Leon to a place like this, and I prefer to keep Sarah away as much as possible too. I like the growing expertise with which I find this place — two left turns, a long corridor, past the elevator banks which took me down to the ward where I had Lemtrada and out across the sloping, creaking walkway between buildings and down, down, down the two flights of stairs. And then sunlight and a row of empty plastic seats opposite a small, wood-grain panelled door.

Except today the seats are not empty. They are filled with other people, and as I sit and listen to their chatting – some of them have brought a friend or a relative, others are merely nodding almost imperceptibly when something is said that they agree with – I realize that all of us, all of us in the corridor, have one thing in common.

And we are so different. We are all clearly at different stages, both of the disease itself and of our understanding of it. I think of the revelation I had in hospital, that I am too eager to look for guides. And yet somehow, even after I met Justine as she was finishing her own course of Lemtrada, I never looked for guides here, among the people who were exploring the same territory as me.

A memory returns as I settle in and wait for my tests. I am suddenly five or six, and packing a huge rucksack with the sorts of things a five- or six-year-old thinks they might need to pack in a rucksack. My mother helps me squeeze into the straps and, as I teeter under the clanking weight of that pack, filled with blankets, toys, bottles, hand-drawn maps, she opens the front door and we head out for the day, out to the park beyond our house to climb a tall hill that has a funny little building at the top of it, bleached white stone surrounded by low railings. As we walk, I warn Mum that the climb is going to be dangerous and tricky. She will probably need to be rescued several times. I hope I am up to it.

And the climb, of course, lasts all of about twelve seconds. Maybe longer when you throw in a little showboating and drama, maybe a whole extra minute once I discover a patch of quicksand, which we both have to get stuck in, one after the other, before finding vines at the last second to pull us clear. A polite, even democratic kind of adventure, all told, everybody getting their moment to shine.

At the summit, I eat a squashed sandwich and suggest that Mum might help carry my rucksack on the way home after I rescued her. And then it comes to me: we should be in a club. We've earned our place today. We deserve a club for this. We could call it the Explorers' Club. We could have membership cards.

Did I make membership cards? Back then, I seemed to make new membership cards almost every week for some venture or another, so I imagine I did. I can almost see them, little fragments of lined paper, covered with blotchy felt-pen lettering. A club of two.

And here, I guess, is a club of more than two. Here is my new Explorers' Club. I share things with these people, more than I would like to admit. A disease, for sure. A few symptoms, undoubtedly. And Quill, I probably share him, with enormous reluctance. And Dr Koenig. And so much more I have not got the energy to list.

I find I am now starting to look at my disease as it is in the world – and that means, shamefully late, looking to other people who have it. New symptoms real and imagined no longer lead me to neurology books but to blogs by fellow patients where I read of the fog that descends unexpectedly, of proprioception problems, of symptoms scattered wherever nerves travel – and nerves must travel everywhere. People often talk of feeling moths on their skin as their eyelids spasm. I have felt these moths. One man can sense his hands but not his arms, so his hands hang in empty space by his side. Some people, far younger than me, developed progressive MS in their late teens and have been bedbound for years – a shutter descends, but a vivid life remains. It is astonishing to see the

extremes of illness MS can inflict, and astonishing to see how
people make a life with the worst of it – and not just make a life,
but reach out to help newcomers like me.

And it is a reminder. At the start of this, I told myself, even
if I would not admit it to others, that I felt like the right person
for the job. I felt that if MS was going to happen to anyone, it
might as well happen to me – who finds the brain interesting,
who is endlessly eager to philosophize about identity, who is
fascinated by disease and the human body and who, perhaps,
has a difficult relationship with reality at the best of times.

But I now see that I was also well suited for this in another
way: I could deal with it. Not emotionally, perhaps. But I could
deal with it in terms of infrastructure, in terms of the frame-
work of privilege that I can now, through my disease, see the
contours of very clearly. I have a comfortable existence, as they
might have said in the nineteenth century. I was able to buy a
house, able to call on nearby family to help look after my child
when needed. I have a job that supports me in my illness. I have
Sarah. I have Leon. I exist in a time when there are treatments
for the disease that I have. And I exist in a country where there's
an NHS, which means I can rely on the kind of expertise I
would never be able to afford in another country. At the start of
this, I did not question that my neurologists were brilliant
people with brilliant training. I assumed it, and I was right to
assume it. I did not question how many astonishing people
were suddenly on my side.

Another trick, then. Another revelation. MS made visible the
nerves beneath the surface of the skin, informed me of the electrical world that makes thought and movement possible. But it
also made visible the accident of good fortune. Is it unfair to get
MS? Not really. Somebody has to get it. The rarefied situation
of comfort from which I get to experience my steady decline,
however? *That* is probably unfair.

And there is one last thing MS has made visible: it has made visible what is at stake. On the bus into town a weekend or so back, Leon suddenly looked at Sarah and said: 'I'm not going to die.'

Sarah and I glanced at each other as we tried to make sense of this. A few stops back, Leon had been telling us she wanted a pink streak in her hair. 'You're not going to dye?' Sarah asked. 'You're not going to dye your hair?'

'No.' Leon frowned. 'I'm not going to die *myself*. I'm not going to die.'

I had been here before, in this sort of conversation, years back at university with a nervous friend who would get panic attacks before lectures when he suddenly realized that he was going to die – not now, but one day, eventually, and this knowledge rendered the moment he was in completely unliveable. I was nineteen probably, and a fool. My response was to lie to him. 'I wouldn't worry,' I would say. 'By the time we get old they will have cured it.' I meant dying.

But here on the bus I could not lie. It would set us off on the wrong footing for ever. I was pondering how to tell the truth, when Sarah did it for us. The nurse in her. Or rather the part of her that made her perfectly suited to being a nurse in the first place.

'Everybody dies, Leon,' said Sarah, putting a hand on Leon's tiny shoulder. 'Everybody dies, just like everybody is born. It is something we all have to do one day, a long way off. And that is all right. And we are all here to talk about it whenever you want to.'

There is something in this that gets to the heart of a worry I have: a worry about where I will be in the future, and what kind of parent I will be able to be in the future. And in this moment I look at Sarah, at how beautifully she is navigating this crucial instance, hugging Leon and meeting her frowning gaze, and I think: I am here *now*, Leon. At least I am here now. And I am learning what it actually means to be here for you.

A week or so ago, I got an Instagram notification: a new account had started following me. Batting aside Mrs Angemi, I stared at the face on the profile of this new account and saw that it was the face of my own brother Ben. And here he is, spread over a handful of snaps: his life in Worcester, and his daughters. Guitar lessons, after-school clubs, homework and Sunday lunches: a life that I feel I understand, even if it is nothing like ours.

In truth, I have always been slow to see things, to understand things. My own privilege. My own good fortune. I was slow to see my daughter clearly, and understand the ultimate link between us – a dreamy man unable to see he had a dreamy child. I saw this far later than Sarah did. But I see it now on a cold morning on the unfinished road outside our house.

After I showed her the pictures of Ben and his children, Leon wanted to write her cousins a letter. As she worked on it at a plastic table set up in the living room, the letter changed.

And so we left home one morning last week with a treasure map. A treasure map that had once been a letter. I hung back a little as she led the way, consulting the spirals and staircases drawn on the map in confident strokes of thick blue pen.

'The map says it's up this way,' she said as we got to the end of our driveway. She stopped again at the end of the bumpy, unfinished road. 'There are going to be hills and down-hills,' she warned me, and then, very seriously, she said: 'We're going to have to walk on *grass*.'

Everything we encountered that morning had been foreseen by the map she held. 'We were supposed to spot that car,' she said as we inched past a red Volvo that had parked on the edge of the kerb. 'We were supposed to see that bird,' she said, as a crow took off for a nearby tree.

We rounded a corner and started up a hill, past a house where a dog was slumped on some steps. Leon looked at her map once more.

'That dog is where I expected it to be,' she said, nodding.

She folded the map and stuck it in a pocket, and we continued up the hill.

Notes on Sources

Since my first consultation with Dr Quill I have been fascinated by the ways that we explore the brain. For the medical profession, there are high-tech options like MRIs and SPECT scans, but to my surprise the low-tech solutions are equally common. I have yet to meet a neurologist who did not want me to close my eyes and reach out with both hands, for example, or who was not interested in timing me as I walked the length of a corridor outside their office.

For the rest of us, books remain the best way in. I have read many books on the brain over the last three or four years, but the book that has had the greatest impact on my thinking is undoubtedly *Mind Wide Open: Why You Are What You Think*, by Steven Johnson (London: Penguin Books, 2004), which I read long before I was diagnosed with MS, back in my early twenties. It was Johnson who first introduced me to Paul MacLean's triune brain theory, and my conception of the brain as a mixologist, skimming me cocktails of neurotransmitters and hormones, always with my well-being in mind, but not always with my consent, is heavily based on my (mis)reading of Johnson's work.

Once I was diagnosed with MS, I was filled with a great curiosity about the brain and the people who had helped bring it into the light over the years. In this regard, I was delighted to find *Minds Behind the Brain: A History of the Pioneers and Their Discoveries*, by Stanley Finger (Oxford: Oxford University Press, 2000): a history of neurology that is firmly focused on the people making the discoveries. Finger's book has been a good friend to me as my illness has progressed, and it remains the primary source for much of my understanding of the history of neurology.

Finger's chapter on Jean-Martin Charcot provided me with my first real introduction to this confusing and contradictory figure, but I have also been influenced by a few other texts. *Charcot: Constructing Neurology*, by Christopher G. Goetz, Michel Bonduelle and Toby Gelfand (Oxford: Oxford University Press, 1995), is a wonderful biography that attempts to put his work on MS in a much wider context, and I am also indebted to the description of Charcot's clinical work in MS – and the work that preceded him – in *Multiple Sclerosis: The History of a Disease*, by T. Jock Murray (New York: Demos, 2005), another central source for this book, covering everything from potential early MS sightings to the last few centuries' ponderings over the potential causes.

In the following pages I have tried to make sense of the rest of my reading. Over the course of writing this book I have also been very lucky to conduct several long interviews with neurologists, exploring everything from the mechanisms behind MS symptoms to the ways that MS patients actually react to their diagnoses. I am enormously grateful for their time. All errors in the text belong to me and me alone.

Epigraph

'When a patient calls on you . . .': Goetz, Bonduelle and Gelfand, *Charcot*, p. 135.

1. The Inland Empire

'*marked enfeeblement* . . .': Jean-Martin Charcot, quoted in Murray, *Multiple Sclerosis*, p. 461.

'that my diagnosis didn't have to be a total disaster . . .': I was almost certainly thinking of *An Anthropologist on Mars*, by Oliver Sacks (London: Picador, 1995), in which he writes, 'Nearly all of my patients, so it seems to me, whatever their problems, reach out to life – and not only despite their conditions, but often because of them . . .', p. xvi.

The Marrow of the Skull

Details of the Edwin Smith Surgical Papyrus and my understanding of Egypt's painful early form of neurology in the Third Dynasty comes from the chapter 'An Ancient Egyptian Physician: The Dawn of Neurology', in Finger, *Minds Behind the Brain*, pp. 7–19.

2. Lost

'with the map at the front followed by illustrations from Mervyn Peake . . .': My sense of Mervyn Peake's illustrations is the result of reading both *Peake's Progress: Selected Writings and Drawings of Mervyn Peake*, by Mervyn Peake and edited by Maeve Gilmore (London: Allen Lane, 1978), and *Vast Alchemies: The Life and Work of Mervyn Peake*, by G. Peter Winnington (London: Peter Owen Publishers, 2000).

The Man Who Couldn't Open a Door

Christine's story is found in 'The Disembodied Lady', in Oliver Sacks, *The Man Who Mistook His Wife for a Hat* (London: Picador, 2007), pp. 47–58.
'I feel my body . . .': ibid., p. 55.

Beyond Sacks's description, my understanding of the mechanisms behind proprioception are based on my own conversations with neurologists.

Phineas Gage, the Most Famous Neurological Patient in History

Few neurological patients have been as widely discussed as Phineas Gage. The details in this chapter are taken from John Fleischman, *Phineas Gage: A Gruesome but True Story about Brain Science* (Boston: Houghton Mifflin, 2002). Tellingly, I feel I may have been drawn to this book because it is clearly aimed at a teenage audience. Regardless, Fleischman's account of Gage's horrific injury is extremely vivid, and he does a wonderful job of placing him within the medical context of his day. I am particularly indebted to his discussion of the argument playing out between the localizers and whole-brainers (pp. 34–42).

The First Recorded Case of MS

MS viewed as a nineteenth-century disease: Finger, *Minds Behind the Brain*, p. 183.

Halldora – written as 'Halla' – is briefly discussed in Murray, *Multiple Sclerosis*, p. 26, while 'The Saga of Bishop Thorlak' can be read here: http://www.vsnrweb-publications.org.uk/Text%20Series/ Thorlaks%20saga.pdf.

St Lidwina is also covered in Murray, *Multiple Sclerosis*, pp. 21–6, and her story is further discussed in Caroline Walker Bynum, *Holy Feast and Holy Fast: The Religious Significance of Food to Medieval Women* (Berkeley: University of California Press, 1987), pp. 124–9.

Augustus d'Este is widely covered in MS literature, but I actually discovered him for the first time several years ago as he was briefly a patient of Sake Dean Mohamed (1759–1851), also known as Dr Brighton. Mohamed is a local hero in Brighton. Born in east India, he travelled to the UK after serving in the army as a trainee surgeon. Besides tending to the sick, he also introduced shampoo to Europe, and opened the first Indian restaurant in England in 1810. D'Este is written about at length in Murray, *Multiple Sclerosis*, pp. 32–41, but it is best to encounter him through his own words. His remarkable diary can be read at: https://www.ncbi.nlm.nih.gov/pmc/articles/PMC1998243/.

5. *The Dead Teach the Living*

'Remember me when I am gone away . . .', Christina Rossetti, 'Remember', in *The Oxford Book of English Verse, 1250–1918*, ed. Sir Arthur Quiller-Couch (London: Clarendon Press, 1939), p. 967.

'I Only Observe, Nothing More'

On the history of the Salpêtrière hospital: Finger, *Minds Behind the Brain*, p. 179; Goetz, Bonduelle and Gelfand, *Charcot*, p. 64.

Picturing Charcot at work: Goetz, Bonduelle and Gelfand, *Charcot*, pp. 137–9; Murray, *Multiple Sclerosis*, p. 126.

Charcot's lectures, held on Tuesdays and Fridays, are the stuff of neurological legend. For a vivid, if unreliable, description of their strange atmosphere, see Axel Munthe, *The Story of San Michele* (1929; London: John Murray, 2004), p. 203.

'above average in his knowledge . . .': Goetz, Bonduelle and Gelfand, *Charcot*, p. 16.

visuel: Sigmund Freud, *Sigmund Freud, Volume III: Early Psychoanalytic Publications* (London: Vintage, 2001), p. 12.

'He was not a reflective man . . .': ibid.

'All I am is a photographer': Goetz, Bonduelle and Gelfand, *Charcot*, p. 90.

'I only observe, nothing more': ibid.

'if you say [a doctor] is . . .': Finger, *Minds Behind the Brain*, p. 177.

On the anatomo-clinical method: Goetz, Bonduelle and Gelfand, *Charcot*, pp. 65–72.

'Years of patient waiting . . .': Freud, *Sigmund Freud, Volume III*, p. 14.

'[Charcot] used to look . . .': ibid., p. 12.

On the doctors who spotted features of MS: Murray, *Multiple Sclerosis*, p. 96.

On tremor and the separation of MS and Parkinson's: Goetz, Bonduelle and Gelfand, *Charcot*, pp. 113–20.

'We are sometimes reproached . . .': ibid., p. 169.

6. The Ghost on the Green

My understanding of diplopia comes from discussions with neurologists.

On the visual cortex: Stephen Macknick and Susana Martinez-Conde, *Sleights of Mind: What the Neuroscience of Magic Reveals about Our Brains* (London: Profile Books, 2011), pp. 11–13.

On the eyes as an extension of the brain: Laura Cumming, *A Face to the World: On Self-Portraits* (London: HarperPress, 2010), p. 28.

On the macula and the fovea: Macknick and Martinez-Conde, *Sleights of Mind*, pp. 29–30.

On creative licence being applied by the visual cortex: ibid., p. 13.

My understanding of Charles Bonnet syndrome is based on my discussions with neurologists.

Myelin, the Mysterious — and Misunderstood — Substance at the Heart of MS

On the discovery of the role the immune system plays in MS: Murray, *Multiple Sclerosis*, pp. 240–41.

On Luigi Galvani's work on the nerves: Finger, *Minds Behind the Brain*, p. 112.

On new discoveries regarding myelin: https://www.newscientist.com/article/mg22530090-600-brain-boosting-its-not-just-grey-matter-that-matters/; my interview with Dr William Richardson.

7. *Hyde*

Laniakea video: https://www.scientificamerican.com/article/laniakea-mapping-laniakea-the-milky-way-s-cosmic-home-video/.

Allan Ropper's book: Allan Ropper and B. D. Burrell, *Reaching Down the Rabbit Hole: Extraordinary Journeys into the Human Brain* (London: Atlantic Books, 2015).

Joan Didion, *The Year of Magical Thinking* (London: Harper Perennial, 2006), p. 47.

Hollowing as a Sacks term: Oliver Sacks, 'The Last Hippie', in *An Anthropologist on Mars* (London: Picador, 1995), p. 41.

Robert Louis Stevenson biography: Claire Harman, *Robert Louis Stevenson: A Biography* (London: Harper Perennial, 2010), p. xvii.

The Viking Gene, the Equator and Vitamin D

On MS being hereditary: https://www.mstrust.org.uk/a-z/risk-developing-ms

On the causes of MS: 'Searching for a Cause of MS', Murray, *Multiple Sclerosis*, pp. 229–318; Charcot's observations: ibid., p. 124;

overworking: ibid., p. 177; too much thinking: ibid., p. 142; sexual habits: ibid., p. 175; toxins: ibid., p. 180.

Charcot on gender imbalance: ibid., p. 122.

The role of geography: ibid., p. 162.

Orkney Islands: https://www.theguardian.com/society/2012/dec/10/orkney-islands-multiple-sclerosis-rate.

8. Inside the Tent

'Who is the third who walks always beside you . . .': T. S. Eliot, *The Waste Land*, in *The Complete Poems and Plays of T. S. Eliot* (London: Faber and Faber, 1969), p. 73.

'place lag': Mark Vanhoenacker, *Skyfaring: A Journey with a Pilot* (London: Vintage, 2015), p. 23.

The Art of Diagnosis

Poor-diagnosis anecdote: Murray, *Multiple Sclerosis*, p. 220.

9. The Explorers' Club

Interview with Adam Platt: https://longform.org/posts/longform-podcast-133-adam-platt.

My thoughts on *Las Meninas* are inevitably influenced by Laura Cumming's brilliant reading of the painting in her *A Face to the World*, pp. 118–33.

'The Schreuderspitze': Mark Helprin, *Ellis Island and Other Stories* (New York: Harcourt, 2005).

Line from Saul Bellow: Saul Bellow, *Humboldt's Gift* (London: Penguin Books, 1975), p. 256.

Acknowledgements

This memoir began life as a book review. It probably would have stayed in that form if not for Helen Lewis and Xan Rice at the *New Statesman*. Many thanks for their intervention, and for the permission to use excerpts from two of my *New Statesman* pieces: 'The Alphabet of Months' and 'A Day Out to an Offshore Wind Farm on a Boat Called *Defiance*'.

My eternal thanks to Sam Copeland and all at RCW, and to Venetia Butterfield, Isabel Wall, Poppy North and everyone at Penguin. Thanks for your patience and generosity and kindness and insight. Thanks to the wonderful Jean Garnett at Little, Brown and to Caroline Pretty, who caught the word 'impedimenta' before I used it incorrectly in print, but agreed that it was a beauty anyway.

Regarding neurological matters, thanks to Dr Omar Hafeez-Bore, Dr Bazo Raheem, Dr Richard Nicholas, Dr William Richardson and Aleksandra Herman. Thanks to David Colhurst and the work of his students. Thanks also to Andrea Lisher, Jenna Mahoney and everyone at the MS Society. All errors in the discussion of brain science in this book are mine and mine alone.

Thanks and love to Simon Parkin, Will Porter and Keith Stuart, to Matt Milne, Nathan Ditum, Pat Tod, Michael Gapper, Michael Cook, Alexis Kennedy, Brian Hampton and to Adam Shaw. Thanks to Jonathan Davis, Stuart Pearce and Alasdair Boreham, to Charles Sabine, Jason Killingsworth, Darren Garrett, Sally Clayton, Nick Sheerin, Joe Skrebels, James Smythe and Craig Owens. Thanks to Andy Farrant and

Rachel Weber. Thanks to all at Failbetter Games and all at Ubisoft Reflections. Thanks to Ken Moffat. Thanks to Gazebo Mondrian.

Thanks and endless admiration to the NHS. Particularly, thanks to Jonathan Knibb, Leonora Fisniku, Nadia Abdo, and Anna, Kate and Giles. Thanks to Jocelyn. Thanks to Waqar Rashid. Thanks to the locum who was certain I had Guillain–Barré syndrome and the registrar who explained very recently that the brisk swooshing noises I sometimes hear in my head might be the sounds of blood flow that we learn to ignore in early childhood, returning suddenly through the intervention of MS.

Thanks to Martin, Oli, Wes, Rupert, Ellie, John, various Chrises, Tom, Bertie, James G., Matt, Aoife, Johnny, Ian, Rich and everyone at the Gamer Network.

Thanks to my glorious and enormous family, in particular my sister Janey. Thanks to Barbara and Gerald Halsey.

Thanks and limitless love to Sarah Lea and Leontine Maple. There are no words for this feeling.

We love stories.

Fact or fiction, long or short, exploring distant lands, imagined worlds or your own back yard – anything can be a story, and every place has stories waiting to be told. And we want to find them.

Do you have a story to tell? Want help cutting through the jargon, answers to your burning questions or advice from top authors, agents and editors across the industry?

Find out more about how to get published at:
www.penguin.co.uk/publishmybook